Series Title: **Emerging Technologies in Women's Health**

Volume Title: Robotic Surgery in Gynecology

Editors

Togas Tulandi
McGill University
Canada

&

Arnold Advincula
University of Central Florida
USA

CONTENTS

FOREWORD

Professor Tulandi has to be congratulated for the present e-book about computer enhanced (robotics) in gynecology. As usual, he is right there in the frontiers of new and exciting developments!

This e-book is a timely and a very comprehensive contribution. Each of the authors is a trailblazer in this new discipline. The well-written chapters will assist the reader in embarking on the use of this fascinating development to help their patients. Any physician or patient interested in this new development will benefit immensely from reading this e-book. I like to congratulate him on this well-done job.

In 1986 and later in 1992, we stated that "wherever in the body a cavity exists or a cavity can be created, operative laparoscopy is indicated and probably preferable…. and that the main limitation to operative laparoscopy is the surgeon's imagination….

Further, we presented the first laparoscopic bowel, bladder, and ureter resection and reanastomosis in video-presentations and abstracts in several meetings in 1989, including the annual meeting of ACOG held in Atlanta, the annual ASRM (previously AFS) meeting held in San Francisco, and the AAGL annual meeting in Washington, D.C. It was not until 2004, that following a randomized study with positive results titled "A comparison of laparoscopically assisted and open colectomy for colon cancer" in the New England Journal of Medicine that the editor of the journal, Dr. Pappas wrote: "Surgeons must progress beyond the traditional techniques of cutting and sewing, to a future in which minimal access to the abdominal cavity are only the beginning". This proclamation came nearly nineteen years after the report of our first reported laparoscopic bowel resection. Today, there is a substantial body of evidence to support that the laparoscopic approach is the preferred method for practically all procedures that previously required laparotomy, including surgery for malignancies.

To date, despite all the proven advantages of minimally invasive surgery, most procedures like hysterectomies and bowel resections are done by laparotomy due to the lack of trained endoscopic surgeons and lack of proper instruments. The advent of computer enhanced technology incorporated into laparoscopic surgery will help in bringing significant changes. The DaVinci Robot developed by pioneer robotic scientists Ajit Shah and Phil Green, is an example of potentials of this technology. This "robot" enables visualization of the surgical field in three dimensions, eliminates tremors, has more wrist motions, and allows a quicker learning curve for suturing. I am certain it will convert more laparotomies to minimally invasive surgery.

This e-book will have a good place in history as it is one-of- a -kind in assisting many surgeons in helping their patients by doing less laparotomies and more minimally invasive surgeries. Congratulations again.

Camran Nezhat
Stanford University Medical Center
USA

PREFACE

Numerous treatments and devices have been introduced into the armamentarium to treat disorders and diseases in women. Due to rapid advances in new technologies, clinicians and researchers are not always updated with their knowledge. Indeed, there are many new technologies in women's health, I have identified many new technologies in women's health. These include robotic surgery, new imaging technologies, novel treatment of uterine fibroid including MR guided focused ultrasound, image capturing, virtual reality and many others. These topics become E-book series on *"Emerging Technologies in Women's Health"*.

The first e-book in this series is *Robotic Surgery in Gynecology* and the guest editor is Dr. Arnold Advincula. Dr. Advincula is a Professor of Obstetrics and Gynecology at the University of Central Florida College of Medicine and a pioneer in Robotic Surgery. The contributors are experts in advanced laparoscopy surgery and robotic surgery. Each chapter contains many illustrations by line drawing, photographs and surgical technique which is illustrated step by step. As the technique is relatively new, we allow overlapping of the chapters allowing the readers to learn different techniques from the experts.

This concise and practical e-book on robotic surgery is for practicing gynecologists, residents of Obstetrics and Gynecology, fellows of Reproductive Endocrinology and fellows of Minimally Invasive Surgery. Readers will gain an understanding of robotic surgery in gynecology, its advantages and disadvantages and learn about the development and delivery of this technique. We also hope that this book will be helpful in directing new investigations and the clinical management of patients.

Togas Tulandi
McGill University,
Canada.

LIST OF CONTRIBUTORS

Arnold P. Advincula, MD, FACOG, FACS

Professor of Obstetrics & Gynecology
University of Central Florida College of Medicine
Medical Director, Gynecologic Robotics
Director, AAGL/SRS Minimally Invasive Surgery Fellowship
Florida Hospital - Celebration Health

Nora Alghothani, MD

Mount Carmel Health Systems
Columbus, Ohio

Shabnam Dadgar, MD

Fellow, Atlanta Center for Special Minimally Invasive Surgery & Reproductive Medicine

Tommaso Falcone, M.D., FRCSC, FACOG

Professor and Chair Obstetrics, Gynecology and Women's Health Institute
Cleveland Clinic
9500 Euclid Ave - A81
Cleveland, Ohio USA, 44195

Rosanne Kho, MD

Assistant Professor
Associate Program Director
Division of Urogynecology and Pelvic Reconstructive Medicine
Department of Gynecologic Surgery
Mayo Clinic Arizona
Phoenix, AZ

Javier F Magrina, MD

Director Gynecologic Oncology
Professor, Obstetrics and Gynecology
Barbara Woodward Lips Professor
Mayo Clinic Arizona
Phoenix, Arizona

Catherine Matthews

Associate Professor and Division Chief of Urognecology and Reconstructive Pelvic Surgery
University of North Carolina, Chapel Hill, NC.

Ceana Nezhat, MD, FACOG, FACS

Chair, Department of Obstetrics & Gynecology, Northside Hospital
Associate Professor of Obstetrics & Gynecology (Adj. Clin.), Stanford University School of Medicine
Clinical Associate Professor of Gynecology & Obstetrics, Emory University School of Medicine
Fellowship Director, Atlanta Center for Special Minimally Invasive Surgery & Reproductive Medicine

Geetu Pahlajani, MD

Research Fellow
Obstetrics, Gynecology and Women's Health Institute

Cleveland Clinic
9500 Euclid Ave - A81
Cleveland, Ohio USA, 44195

Sejal Dharia Patel, MD
Center for Reproductive Medicine
3435 Pinehurst Ave, Orlando, FL 32803
Michael C. Pitter, MD, FACOG
Chief of Gynecological Robotic & Minimally Invasive Surgery
Newark Beth Israel Medical Center
201 Lyons Avenue,
Newark, New Jersey USA 07112
Telephone: (973)926-4600
Facsimile: (973)926-4601
Email: mail@drpitter.net

Vanna Zanagnolo, MD
Deputy Director
Division of Gynecology
European Institute of Oncology
Milan, Italy

2

CHAPTER 1

Robot-Assisted Laparoscopy: Basic Principles, Equipment, and Instrumentation

Arnold P. Advincula*

Professor of Obstetrics & Gynecology, University of Central Florida College of Medicine, Medical Director of Gynecologic Robotics, Global Robotics Institute, Director of Minimally Invasive Surgery Fellowship, Florida Hospital – Celebration Health, 410 Celebration Place, Suite 302, Celebration, FL 34747

Abstract: Advancements in conventional laparoscopy have allowed surgeons to treat more surgical pathology in a minimally invasive fashion. However, many procedures are still performed predominantly by laparotomy. Conventional laparoscopic instrumentation and the steep learning curve are often cited as possible obstacles to minimally invasive surgery. The advent and evolution of robotic technology may provide means to overcome the limitations seen with conventional laparoscopy through the use of three-dimensional imaging and more dexterous and precise instruments.

ROBOTICS IN GYNECOLOGY – INTRODUCTION

Historically, surgery in gynecology has been accomplished through a laparotomy or vaginal approach. The laparotomy approach may seem advantageous for the surgeon as a result of depth perception and tactile feedback from tissue. However, the large abdominal incision, prolonged hospitalization, increased postoperative analgesic requirements, and increased morbidity are disadvantages for the patient. The days of a surgeon obtaining access to the abdomen by laparotomy only have long passed. Studies have clearly shown that laparoscopic surgery allows faster recovery with shorter hospitalization, cosmetically better, decreased blood loss and less postoperative pain [1-3].

Technical advancements have brought about improvements to modern day laparoscopy. These include multi-chip cameras and high intensity light sources as well as improved hand instrumentation and energized devices. This technology has continued to grow by leaps and bounds in the area of minimally invasive gynecologic surgery. Despite these technological advancements and proven benefits, some surgeons are still performing laparotomy for complex procedures such as the management of advanced endometriosis, and for procedures that require extensive suturing such as myomectomy and sacrocolpopexy.

A major obstacle to the more widespread acceptance and application of minimally invasive surgical techniques to gynecologic surgery has been the steep learning curve for the surgeons. Other limitations encountered with conventional laparoscopy include counter-intuitive hand movement [fulcrum effect], an unsteady two-dimensional visual field, and limited degrees of instrument motion within the body as well as poor ergonomics and tremor amplification [3]. In an attempt to overcome these obstacles, robotics has been incorporated into the gynecologic armamentarium as a promising solution. The following chapter will provide a brief overview of the history of robotics followed by the current state of equipment and instrumentation.

HISTORY OF ROBOTICS

The concept of robots date back to as early as 1495 when Leonardo da Vinci developed a mechanical armored knight used to amuse royalty. Although other examples of early robots exist in history, it was not until the early 1900s that the concept of robotics entered the popular consciousness. Playwright Karel Capek first coined the term "robot" in 1920 in his satirical drama *Rossum's Universal Robots*. He derived the word robot from the Czech rabota, meaning serf or laborer.

Through the years, robots evolved into a variety of applications including the automobile industry deep sea and space exploration, industrial tasks, and entertainment. The first example of robotics entering the medical field was in 1985.

*Address correspondence to Arnold P. Advincula:** Professor of Obstetrics & Gynecology, University of Central Florida College of Medicine, Medical Director of Gynecologic Robotics, Global Robotics Institute, Director of Minimally Invasive Surgery Fellowship, Florida Hospital – Celebration Health, 410 Celebration Place, Suite 302, Celebration, FL 34747, 407-303-4033; Email: arnold.advincula.md@flhosp.org

A robotic arm was modified to perform a stereotactic brain biopsy with 0.05 mm accuracy [4]. The original model, known as the PUMA 560, was used for neurosurgical stereotactic maneuvers under computed tomography [CT] guidance. In a similar fashion, orthopedic surgery began utilizing a device called ROBODOC in 1992 to perform total hip replacements [5]. The surgeon supplied the dimensions and measurements based on pre-surgical images while the ROBODOC performed the procedure based on that information. A common theme to these early designs was the way in which the robots functioned. They were developed to function autonomously with a preoperative plan or in a supervisory role.

Subsequently, robotics evolved from a passive to a more active role. The concept of robotic telepresence technology was born initially through the collaborative efforts of the Stanford Research Institute [SRI], the Department of Defense, and the National Aeronautics and Space Administration [NASA] [7]. The impetus for this concept was the need to provide remote surgery to wounded soldiers on the battlefield. Initial prototypes involved robotic arms that could be mounted on an armored vehicle in order to facilitate this concept. Soon thereafter, this technology became commercialized and robots were no longer just passive devices in surgery but ones that could be actively controlled in civilian operating rooms. Although robotic telepresence technology was initially created for cardiac surgery [6], its application to the field of gynecology was then followed.

EVOLUTION OF ROBOTS IN MEDICINE

HERMES™ & AESOP®

The first attempt to increase surgeon's control in an automated way over the surgical field was a voice-activated system designed and developed by Computer Motion, Inc. [Goleta, CA]. HERMES™ was a system that used voice recognition to control the laparoscopic camera, light source, insufflation, printer, phone, operating room lights, and patient table position [7]. Soon this technology was combined with one of the early predecessors and first applications of robotic technology in surgery, the automated endoscopic system for optimal position [AESOP®, Computer Motion Inc., Goleta, CA].

In 1994, AESOP® was the first surgical robot to be FDA approved. Designed to reduce surgeon fatigue and offer a stable visual field by controlling the camera during laparoscopy, this active robotic device had motorized joints that were voice activated through the HERMES™ speech recognition program [7, 8]. Gynecologists played an early role in the evaluation of this technology. One study by Mettler *et al.* compared the system to a surgical assistant holding the laparoscope during gynecologic surgery [9]. The authors found that the time required to perform the laparoscopy was faster with the robotic camera holder because it improved efficiency by allowing the two surgeons to use both hands for operating, just as they would in a laparotomy.

ZEUS™

Under the direction of the same company, AESOP® evolved into the Zeus™ surgical system with the addition of two robotic arms. Although originally developed in 1999 for cardiac operations, the Zeus™ minimally invasive surgical robot system later received FDA-approval for its use in laparoscopic surgery in 2001. Dr. Yulan Wang, one of the pioneering forces behind the design of the Zeus® robotic system outlined five essential features for a successful surgical robotic system: multiple robotic arms, improved ergonomics, enhanced dexterity of motion to eliminate intention tremors, high magnification of the surgical field and finally, fast and reliable data transmission between the surgeon and his or her tools and imaging systems.

Constructed as a master-slave device, this two component system consisted of a master console where the surgeon sat comfortably and directed the slave robotic instruments. At the console, the surgeon controlled the robotic arms by maneuvering two joysticks that fit in the palm of the hands while viewing a flat video monitor. In order to achieve three-dimensional visualization, specialized glasses were worn by the surgeon [7, 10]. Through a computer interface, tremors were eliminated as the surgeon's hand movements were downscaled over a range of 2:1 to 10:1 [11].

Three remotely controlled robotic arms were mounted to the operating table. These robotic arms operated the camera in a manner similar to AESOP® but also provided the surgeon with two operating arms that possessed interchangeable "microwrist" instruments that more closely mimic the movements of the human wrist when compared to conventional laparoscopic instruments. The potential axes of motion of the surgical instruments were called "degrees of freedom," of which there are seven: 1) in and out movement, 2) axial rotation, 3) opening and closing the instrument, 4) lateral movement at the articulation, 5) vertical movement at the articulation, 6) left movement at each articulation, 7) right movement at each articulation. This early robotic system represented a significant paradigm shift that placed the surgeon at a remote console instead of standing at the patient's bedside. This ground-breaking concept would be carried into future designs and truly represented telesurgery which defined broadly as the ability to perform surgery from a distance.

Historically, the Zeus™ surgical system became the first robotic device to truly test this concept [13]. In a 45 minute operation entitled "Lindbergh"; surgeons in New York successfully performed a laparoscopic cholecystectomy on a patient located in Strasbourg, France in 2001. This was accomplished with only a time delay of less than 200ms between the controls in New York and the action of the instruments on the patient in Strasbourg, France. Two communication systems were utilized to link both the video feed as well as a telephone link by a fiber optic service [12-14].

Two years later, one of the first remote telesurgical services was designed in Canada in 2003. Anvari and colleagues created a program by which the Zeus™ surgical system was set up in Hamilton, Ontario for the surgeon and the robotic arms were positioned on the patient in North Bay, Ontario – 400km away. They were able to utilize a pre-established commercial network as a communication link between the two locations. Twenty-one laparoscopic surgeries including fundoplications, sigmoid resections, and hemicolectomies were completed successfully with this set-up. The two surgeons on either end were able to operate simultaneously with little time delay for communication and signal reception. They reported no significant complications [15]. Although the feasibility of long distance telesurgery has been proven, costs remain a significant issue along with the inconsistency and unreliability of information transfer over long distances.

Interestingly, there were early studies in the gynecologic arena that reported on the Zeus™ surgical system's successful application to tubal reanastomosis. In one prospective study, pregnancy rates were evaluated in ten patients with previous tubal ligations who underwent laparoscopic tubal reanastomosis using the identical technique used at laparotomy [16]. A post-operative tubal patency rate of 89% was demonstrated in 17 of the 19 tubes anastomosed with a pregnancy rate of 50% at one year. There were no complications or ectopic pregnancies.

Socrates™

During the same time period as that of Zeus™, the FDA also approved Socrates™ [Computer Motion, Inc., Goleta, CA], a robotic telecollaboration device that facilitated telementoring. The telementor from a remote site used this program to connect with an operating room and share audio-visual signals. A key feature of this technology was a telestrator that could annotate anatomy or surgical instructions and a voice controlled system that could control camera movement and other electronic equipment in the distant operating room [17].

Da Vinci® Surgical System

Today's platform of surgical robotics revolves around the daVinci® surgical system [Intuitive Surgical®, Sunnyvale, CA] which is the only actively produced and FDA approved robotic telesurgical system. Intuitive Surgical Inc. acquired Computer Motion, Inc. in 2003 and subsequently phased out the Zeus™ surgical system [10].

Similar to its predecessor, the daVinci® surgical system is comprised of three components which have undergone various modifications over the last decade. The first component is the surgeon console where the surgeon controls the robotic system remotely. The console contains large microcomputer motherboards that direct the movement of the robotic arms. A stereoscopic viewer as well as hand and foot controls is housed in this unit. Seated at the console, the surgeon obtains a binocular view of the surgical field through the stereoscopic viewer while maneuvering both hand and foot controls simultaneously. The stereoscopic viewer also has an infrared sensor which deactivates the robotic arms whenever the surgeon moves his or her head out of the console [18].

Foot pedals located at the base of the console facilitate various functions including: positioning of the camera, focus adjustment, activation of monopolar or bipolar energy sources, repositioning of the handgrips *via* a clutch mechanism, and toggling between instruments [a feature specific to the use of four robotic arms]. The console also adjusts to the surgeon's body habitus for improved ergonomics. The most recent daVinci® surgical system model allows the option of two surgeon consoles to communicate with each other simultaneously during an operative case Fig: **1**.

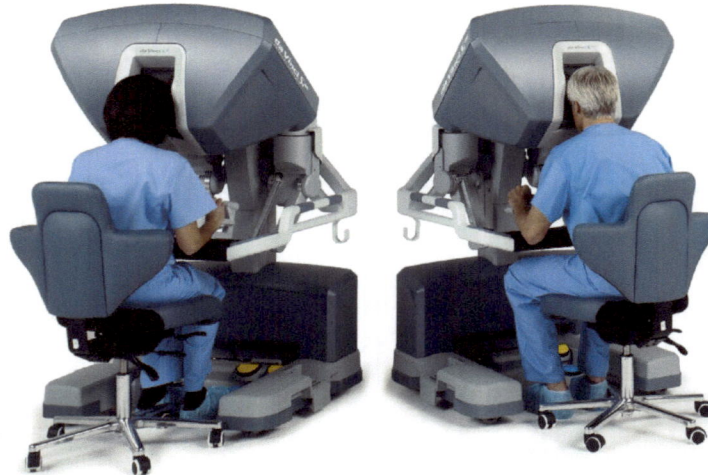

Figure 1: Dual Surgeon Console. Photo courtesy of Intuitive Surgical®.

The second component of the daVinci® surgical system is the InSite® vision system which provides the three dimensional stereoscopic imaging through either an 8.5 mm or 12 mm endoscope Fig. **2**. Because the endoscope of the daVinci® surgical system is composed of two parallel telescopes [0- or 30- degree lenses] which are each capable of sending individual images to the camera head, a three dimensional view of the surgical field is seen at the console as the two images are merged by a computer. The video system provides 10x – 15x magnification as well as high definition.

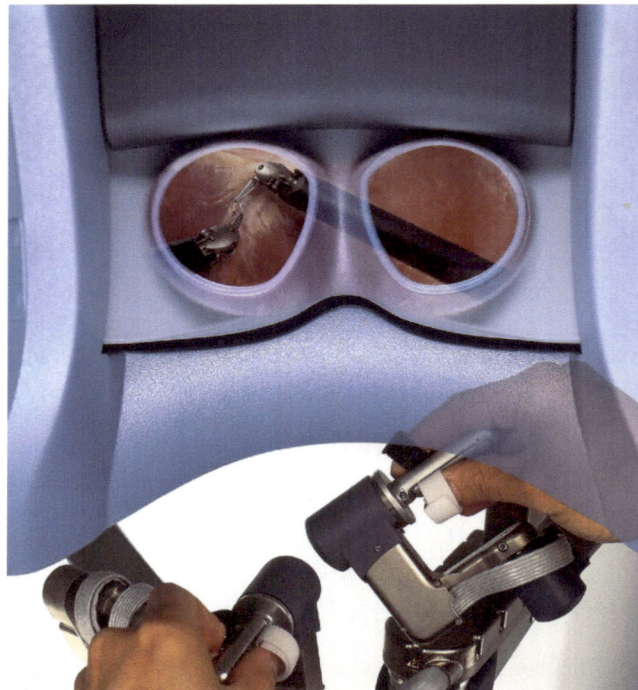

Figure 2: 12 mm InSite® vision system endoscope. Photo courtesy of Intuitive Surgical®.

The third component of the daVinci® surgical system is the patient-side cart with Endowrist® instruments and either three or four robotic arms Fig. **3**. One of the arms holds the laparoscope while the other two t o three arms hold the various interchangeable Endowrist® instruments which come in either 5 mm or 8 mm Fig. **4**. Each grasping instrument has its own preprogrammed maximum pressure and can be used for up to ten cases before being replaced [7, 10]. These surgical instruments also overcome the fulcrum effect of conventional laparoscopy through the seven degrees of freedom described earlier which replicate the full wrist-like motion of the surgeon's hand.

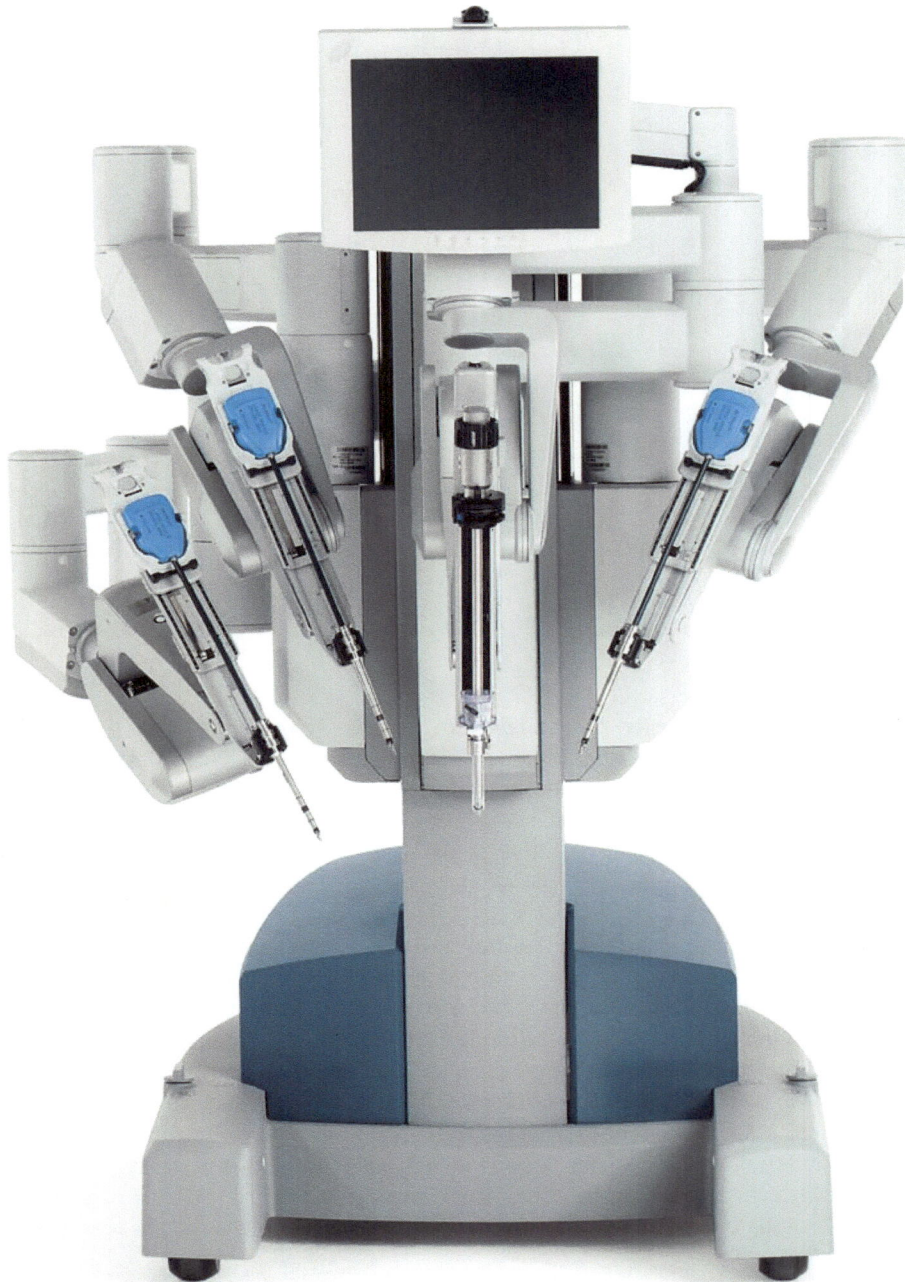

Figure 3: Patient-side cart with four robotic arms. Photo courtesy of Intuitive Surgical®.

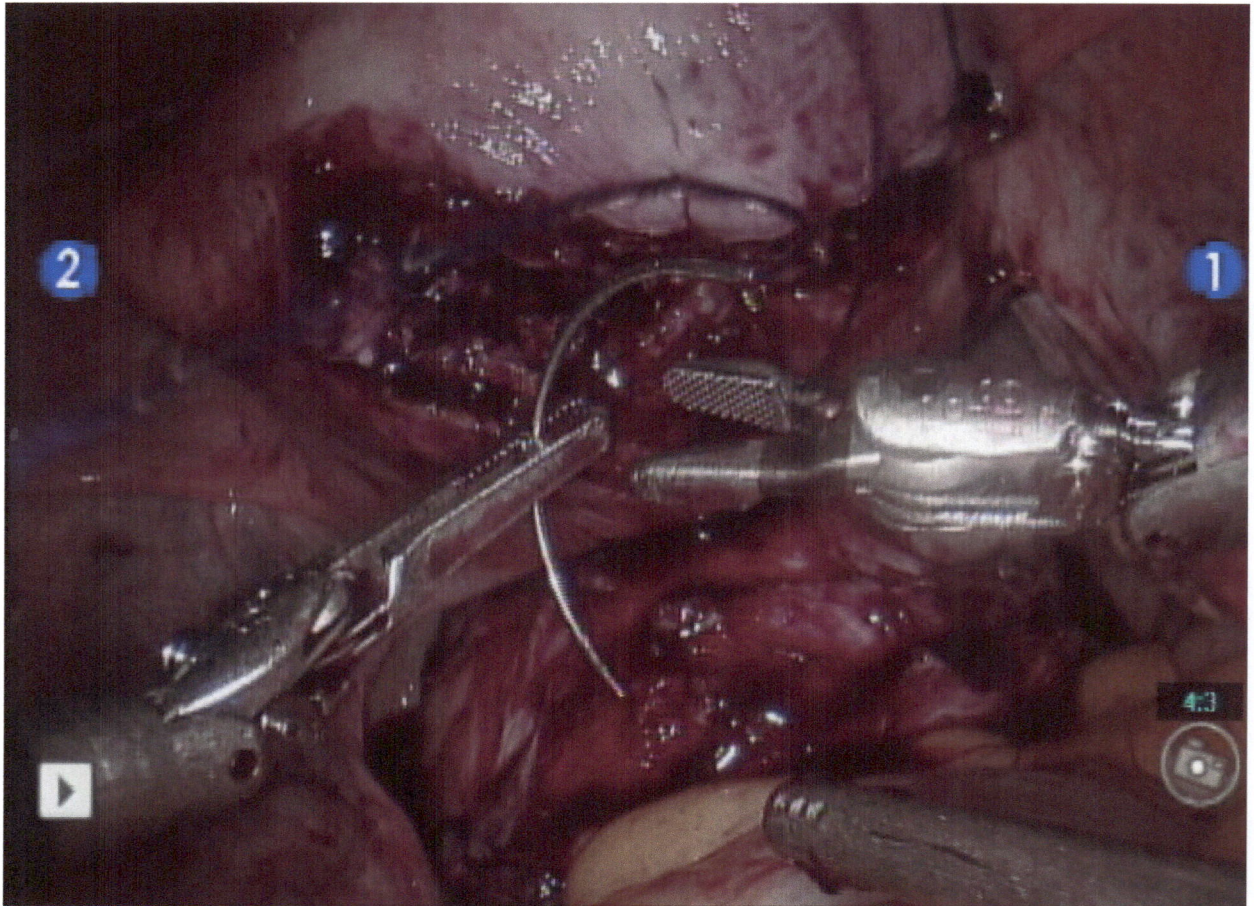

Figure 4: Endowrist(r) instruments.

A wide range of laparoscopic instruments are available such as needle drivers, Debakey forceps, and tenaculum forceps in addition to energized monopolar and bipolar instruments that are placed through specific trocars [18]. These instruments enable the surgeon to manipulate, coagulate, dissect, retract, and suture. This system also allows a greater variety of scaled motion for precise and accurate control [5:1, 3:1, or 1:1] while eliminating tremors [7, 10, 19]. Although articulation is greatly enhanced, there is an absence of haptic (tactile) feedback to the surgeon manipulating the instruments.

Three models currently exist, the original daVinci® Surgical System (known as the Standard), the S-System which was released in 2006, and most recently the Si-System which was released in 2009. Modifications of the original system includes the addition of a fourth surgical arm, longer instruments, increased variety in 5mm or 8mm instruments, an interactive video display, motorized side cart, high definition viewing, and a more streamlined design [10]. The Si-System incorporates an optional dual console which truly allows two surgeons to be simultaneously immersed in a telepresence environment while facilitating surgery in either a collaborative or student-teacher relationship. Manipulation of the hand and foot controls can be shared or transferred back and forth at the discretion of the primary operator. The interactive video display on the two newest models provides the ability to telestrate. An additional feature found on the two newest models is TilePro®. Panels of images such as patient vital signs or radiologic imaging can be integrated into the operative view of the surgeon seated at the console.

Robotic technology has clearly undergone a rapid evolution over the last decade and as with any new technology, careful consideration must be made before incorporating it into one's surgical practice. First and foremost, having a strong rationale for its use is critical. One such reason may be to allow the laparoscopic approach to be more closely modeled after tried and true open surgical techniques thereby making comparisons of surgical outcomes more accurate.

Additionally, robotics may allow not only for more complex cases to be done in a minimally invasive fashion but also cases done by laparotomy to be converted to laparoscopy. In fact, robotics has been shown in numerous studies to be an enabling technology that can shorten learning curves and level the playing field between the novice and expert surgeon thereby potentially facilitating this transition [20]. Most importantly, this technology should not be a replacement for something already done extremely well. Instead it should be viewed as a powerful tool in one's surgical armamentarium that can potentially provide new options for both the patient and surgeon.

Although a solid rationale behind the use of any new technology is important, surgeons must also look at their individual practices to see if the case volume and comfort level is there to tackle the learning curve associated with robotics. As enabling as it may be, robotics is not a surgical approach one can dabble in. Commitment and consistency are keys to successful implementation. Technology cannot be a replacement for sound judgment and a solid understanding of anatomy and the principles of laparoscopic surgery. With all that being said, the current state of robotic technology has already impacted technical approaches and clinical outcomes in gynecologic surgery. The following chapters in this e-book will discuss these revolutionary changes.

ACKNOWLEDGEMENT

Reproduced images should be accompanied by the following copyright notice: ©*[year] Intuitive Surgical, Inc.*

BIBLIOGRAPHIES

[1]   Yuen PM, Yu KM, Yip SK, Lau WC, Rogers MS, Chang A. A randomized prospective study of laparoscopy and laparotomy in the management of benign ovarian masses. Am J Obstet Gynecol 1997; 177: 109-114.

[2]   Lo L, Pun TC, Chan S. Tubal ectopic pregnancy: an evaluation of laparoscopic surgery versus laparotomy in 614 patients. Aust New Zeal J Obstet Gynecol 1999; 39: 185-187.

[3]   Stylopoulos N, Rattner D. Robotics and ergonomics. Surg Clin N Am 2003; 83: 1-12.

[4]   Kwoh YS, Hou J, Jonckheere EA, Hayati S. A robot with improved absolute positioning accuracy for CT guided stereotactic brain surgery. IEEE Trans Biomed Eng 1988; 35: 153-160.

[5]   Bauer A, Borner M, Lahmer A. Clinical experience with a medical robotic system for total hip replacement. In: Nolte LP, Ganz R, eds. Computer assisted orthopedic surgery. Bern: Hogrefe & Huber, 1999; 128-133.

[6]   Diodato MD, Damiano RJ. Robotic cardiac surgery: overview. Surg Clin N Am 2003; 83: 1-12.

[7]   Talamini MA. Robotic surgery: is it for you? Adv Surg 2002; 36: 1-13.

[8]   Marescaux J, Rubino F. The ZEUS robotic system: experimental and clinical applications. Surg Clin North Am 2003; 83: 1305-1315.

[9]   Mettler L, Ibrahim M, Jonat W. One year of experience working with the aid of a robotic assistant [the voice-controlled optic holder AESOP] in gynecologic endoscopic surgery. Hum Reprod 1998; 13: 2748-2750.

[10]   Hockstein, NG, Gourin CG, and Faust RA, Terris DJ. A history of robots: from science fiction to surgical robotics. J Robotic Surg 2007, 1: 113-118.

[11]   Advincula AP, Falcone T. Laparoscopic robotic gynecologic surgery. Obstet Gynecol Clin North Am 2004; 31: 599-609.

[12]   Pande RU, Patle Y, Powers CP, *et al.* The Telecommunication Revolution in the Medical Field: Present Applications and Future Perspective. Curr Surg 2003; 6: 636-640.

[13]   Marecaux J, Leroy J, Gagner M. Transatlantic robotic-assisted telesurgery. Nature 2001; 413: 379-380.

[14]   Marescaux J, Leroy J, Rubino F, *et al.* Transcontinental robot-assisted remote telesurgery: feasibility and potential applications. Ann Surg 2002; 235: 487-492.

[15]   Anvari M, McKinley C, Stein H. Establishment of the world's first telerobotic remote surgical suite. Ann Surg 2005; 241: 460-464.

[16]   Falcone T, Goldberg JM, Margossian H, Stevens L. Robotically assisted laparoscopic microsurgical anastomosis: a human pilot study. Fertil Steril 2000; 73: 1040-1042.

[17]   Ballantyne GH. Robotic surgery, telerobotic surgery, telepresence, and telementoring. Review of early clinical results. Surg Endosc 2002; 16: 1389-402.

[18]   Dharia, SP, Falcone, T. Robotics in reproductive Medicine. Fertil Steril 2005; 84: 1-11.

[19]   Kim HL, and Schulam, P. The PAKY, HERMES, AESOP, ZEUS, and daVinci robotic systems. Urol Clin N Am 2004; 31: 659-669.

[20]   Sarle R, Tewari A, Shrivastava A, Peabody J, Menon M. Surgical robotics and laparoscopic training drills. J Endouro 2004; 18: 63-67.

CHAPTER 2

Robot-Assisted Laparoscopic Colpo- and Cervicosacropexy with the Da Vinci® Surgical System

Catherine A. Matthews*

University of North Carolina, Chapel Hill, NC

Abstract: Abdominal sacrocolpopexy has been considered the gold-standard surgical procedure for repair of apical vaginal support defects. While it is feasible to perform this operation using conventional laparoscopic techniques, a limited number of surgeons have mastered the advanced minimally-invasive skills that are required. Introduction of the da Vinci® robotic system with instruments that have improved dexterity and precision and a camera system with three-dimensional imaging presents an opportunity for more surgeons treating women with pelvic organ prolapse to perform the procedure laparoscopically. This chapter will outline a technique that is exactly modeled after the open procedure for completion of a robotic-assisted colpo- and cervicosacropexy using the da Vinci® surgical system.

INTRODUCTION

The rapid growth of the aging population and high projected prevalence rates of pelvic floor disorders over the next several decades [1,2] presents a formidable need to identify a reconstructive procedure that maximizes efficacy, minimizes risk, and has the lowest interference in normal daily function during the postoperative period. Pelvic organ prolapse (POP) often involves a combination of support defects involving the anterior, posterior, and apical vaginal segments with increasing evidence that the apex presents the cornerstone of pelvic support.[3-5] Abdominal sacrocolpopexy (ASCP) has been considered the gold standard surgical procedure for repair of Level I pelvic support defects. Systemic reviews of mean reoperation rates following sacral colpopexy range from 2.3% [6] to 4.4% [7]. A Cochrane Database review noted ASCP to be associated with a lower rate of recurrent vault prolapse and dyspareunia than vaginal sacrospinous colpopexy. Operative morbidity and length of recovery, however, were higher in the ACSP group [8].

While a small number of surgeons are able to accomplish sacrocolpopexies using standard laparoscopic techniques, the majority are performed *via* laparotomy because of challenges encountered with extensive suturing and knot-tying. Small case series have demonstrated similar outcomes using a laparoscopic approach with the additional benefits of reduced pain, postoperative time for recovery, and length of hospital stay [9-11].

With the introduction of the da Vinci® robot, the feasibility of more surgeons performing this operation through a minimally-invasive technique has greatly expanded. The steep learning curve that is inherent in mastering intracorporeal knot tying and suturing using standard laparoscopy is greatly diminished by the use of articulating instruments, making it an accessible option for all gynecologic surgeons treating women with pelvic organ prolapse. In this chapter we will describe the steps involved in completing a robotic-assisted SCP utilizing a y-shaped polypropylene mesh graft.

SURGICAL PREPARATION AND SET-UP

While evidence-based studies do not support the use of bowel preparations in patients undergoing laparoscopic surgery [12], we instruct patients to drink 2 bottles of magnesium citrate and clear liquids one day prior to surgery as we have found that sigmoid decompression aids in the ability to retract the bowel and expose the sacral promontory. Perioperative antibiotics are administered 30 minutes prior to the procedure and 5000 units of subcutaneous heparin are injected en route to the operating suite for thromboprophylaxis. Patients are placed in the dorsal lithotomy position in Allen stirrups with the buttocks extending one inch over the end of an operating table. To prevent

*Address correspondence to Catherine A. Matthews:** Division of Urogynecology and Reconstructive Pelvic Surgery, University of North Carolina, Chapel Hill, NC 27599; Tel: 919-843-7908; E-mail: Catherine_matthews@med.unc.edu

Togas Tulandi and Arnold Advincula (Eds)

slippage in steep Trendelenburg position, patients are placed directly on egg-crate foam with an additional piece of foam positioned across the upper chest and tightly secured to the bed with a long piece of silk tape. Padded shoulder blocks may also be used with careful placement over the acromioclavicular junction bilaterally as direct pressure over the clavicles may result in a brachial plexus injury [13]. Prior to draping the patient, a table tilt test is performed to ensure that steep trendelenburg can be tolerated by assessing airway pressures, as well as to confirm the patient is safely secured to the bed with no movement. This is an essential step as displacement of the buttocks from the end of the table can dramatically limit the manipulation of instruments placed into the vagina and rectum to assist with dissection and suturing. After the patient is prepped and draped, a foley catheter is placed into the bladder and EEA sizers are inserted into the vagina and rectum. A surgical assistant is seated between the legs to provide adequate vaginal and rectal manipulation during the case.

In the event of any prior abdominal surgery, left upper-quadrant entry is preferred to reduce the risk of bowel injury. Pneumoperitoneum is obtained with a Veress needle technique followed by placement of five trocars (Fig. **1**). Careful port placement is integral to the success of this procedure because 1) Inadequate distances between robotic arms and the camera results in arm collisions and interference, 2) Easy visualization and access to the sacral promontory may be compromised if one inserts the camera too low on the anterior abdominal wall and 3) If the fourth arm is not at least 3 cm above the anterior superior iliac crest (ASIS), successful bowel retraction may be compromised. When evaluating the abdomen prior to trocar insertion, we have determined that at least 15 cm is required between the pubic bone and the umbilicus to rely on this landmark for the 12-mm camera port. If this distance is shorter, as it is in many obese women, then insertion above the umbilicus is necessary.[14] An accessory 12 mm port, used for introduction of sutures and the mesh graft, is placed approximately 10 cm lateral and 4 cm cephalad to the camera in the right upper quadrant. An 8mm robotic port is placed in the right lower quadrant 10 cm lateral to the accessory port and approximately 3 cm above the ASIS. The third and fourth robotic arms are placed 10 cm apart in the left lower quadrant, with the fourth arm typically as far lateral as possible.

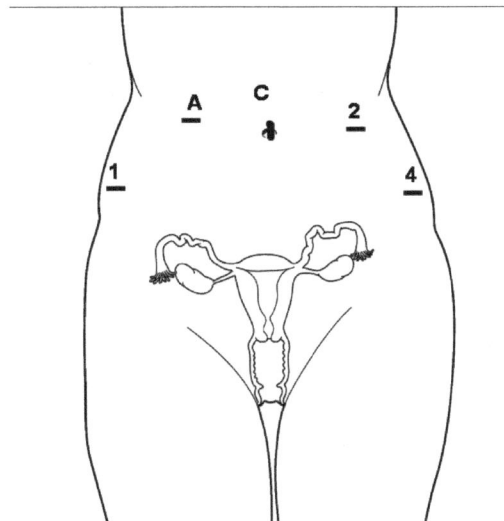

Figure 1: Port placement C= Camera; A= Accessory Port; 1= Right arm (monopolar shears); 2= Left arm (PK Dissector; 3= Fourth Arm (Cadiere Bowel Retractor).

After placing the patient in steep trendelenburg position and locking the bed, the robot is docked from the patient's left side at a 45-degree angle to the bed. Side-docking permits easy access to the vagina for evaluation of graft tension and for completion of cystoscopy to ensure ureteral and bladder integrity. Care should be taken to ensure that the spine of the robot is positioned right next to the bed below the level of the patient's hip as driving it up too high relative to the abdomen can compromise mobility of the fourth arm. In addition, if the robot is not close enough to the bed, reach of the first (right) arm may be limited. Before starting the procedure, it is critical to ensure that the bowel is not obscuring the operative field and efforts to correct this at the beginning of the case can minimize frustration. Monopolar scissors are introduced through the right arm, a bipolar PK™ dissector through the left arm, and an atraumatic bowel grasper such as a cadiere™ is placed through the fourth arm.

ROBOT-ASSISTED LAPAROSCOPIC COLPOSACROPEXY TECHNIQUE

An approach that is exactly modeled after the open surgical technique is critical to the success of a robot-assisted laparoscopic approach to SCP. A bedside assistant is positioned on the patient's right side and the small bowel is moved into the upper abdomen. A fan retractor may assist with retraction if the colon is redundant. With the use of a zero degree scope, the sigmoid colon is retracted to the left side of the abdomen using the cadiere™ forceps which should result in exposure of the sacral promontory. Before opening the peritoneum, the common iliac vessels and the right ureter must be identified. When first attempting this procedure, it may be helpful to identify the sacral promontory with the use of a standard laparoscopic instrument with haptic feedback prior to docking the robot. The peritoneum overlying the sacral promontory is elevated and opened using monopolar cautery. The fat pad overlying the anterior longitudinal ligament is exposed and gently dissected away (Fig. **2**). It is best to direct the tips of the PK dissector and the scissors down to the level of the ligament before bluntly separating the tissue. The middle sacral artery is frequently visualized and can be coagulated using the PK™ dissector if necessary. Care must be exercised to remain in the midline over the sacral promontory as deviation to the left can result in injury to the left iliac vein.

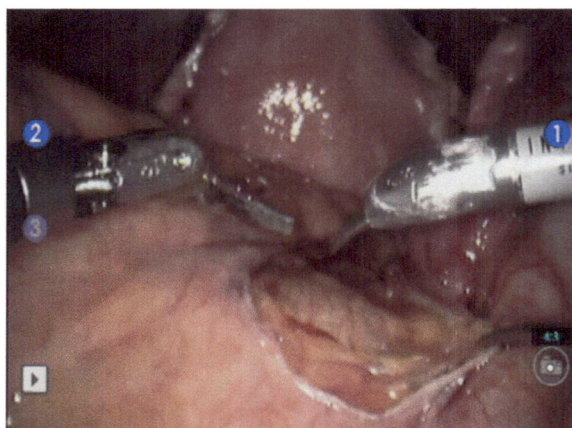

Figure 2: Peritoneum opened at sacral promontory and fat pad dissected to reveal the anterior longitudinal ligament.

A retroperitoneal tunnel is then made from the level of the promontory, along the right paracolic gutter, to the posterior vaginal wall using the scissors and PK dissector. If the tunnel is made just below the peritoneum, all bleeding is avoided and time is saved at the end of the procedure for reperitonealization. With the vagina deviated anteriorly and the rectum posteriorly using the EEA sizers, the rectovaginal space is easily identified and the peritoneal incision is extended transversely in the shape of a "T" to expose the posterior vaginal wall (Fig. **3**). If indicated, the rectovaginal space can be dissected all the way down to the perineal body.

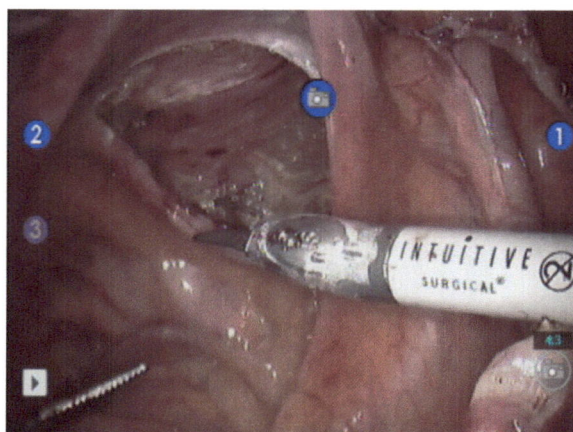

Figure 3: Peritoneal incision is extended along the cul-de-sac to the posterior vaginal wall in a T-shaped configuration to access the rectovaginal space. When performing a cervicosacropexy, it is easiest to develop this surgical plane prior to amputation of the cervix.

The vagina is then deviated posteriorly to facilitate dissection of the bladder from the anterior vaginal wall using monopolar cautery. If significant scarring between the bladder and vagina is encountered, the bladder can be retrograde filled with 300 ml of saline mixed with methylene blue dye to help identify the surgical plane. Depending on the degree of anterior vaginal wall prolapse, approximately 4-6 cm of anterior vaginal wall is exposed. An attempt is made to leave the peritoneum intact at the apex of the vagina to reduce the chance of mesh erosion.

After measuring the respective lengths of the exposed anterior and posterior vaginal walls, a correctly sized y-shaped polypropylene graft is created by suturing together two strips of gynemesh™ that are approximately 3cm in width. Only one arm of the mesh is taken up to the sacrum. Significant variability in the relative dimensions of the anterior and posterior segments of mesh can exist hence the recommendation to fashion the graft after completing the dissection. A pre-sewn polypropylene y-mesh is also commercially available (Intepro ™, American Medical Systems, Minneapolis) and can be cut to fit the vaginal dimensions as well. The only drawback of this mesh is the inability to make it wider in the event of a more capacious vagina.

The mesh graft is introduced through the accessory port after exchanging the scissors and PK dissector for a suture cut and a large needle driver. The bladder is retracted using the fourth arm, and the anterior mesh arm is placed over the anterior vaginal wall and is sutured in place using 2-0 Gore-Tex® sutures on CT-2 needles that are each cut to six inches long. Preliminary data regarding the use of delayed absorbable monofilament suture for mesh attachment suggest that equivalent results, without the risk of suture erosion, are achieved. It is most efficient to anchor the two distal corners first (Figs. **4** and **5**), and then place a series of interrupted stitches towards the vaginal apex (Fig. **6**). The number of sutures required depends on the length of mesh. Knots are tied using two surgeons knots, followed by 2 half-hitches. An attempt is made to achieve healthy bites through the vaginal muscularis without perforating the epithelium. After adequately securing the anterior mesh arm, the vagina is deviated anteriorly and the posterior mesh arm is draped over the posterior vaginal wall with the assistance of the fourth robotic arm which can hold upward traction on the sacral end of the mesh graft. Starting at the vaginal apex, 6-8 interrupted sutures are placed to secure the mesh to the posterior vaginal wall (Fig. **7**). Posterior mesh attachement can be challenging if the vaginal assistant is not providing adequate anterior deviation of the vagina. When suturing in the vertical plane on tissue that is directly infront of the camera, it is easiest to start with the "thumb up" and rotate in a clockwise direction to achieve a healthy bite through the mesh and posterior vaginal wall. If necessary, the zero-degree scope can be exchanged for a 30-degree up-scope to fully visualize the rectovaginal space.

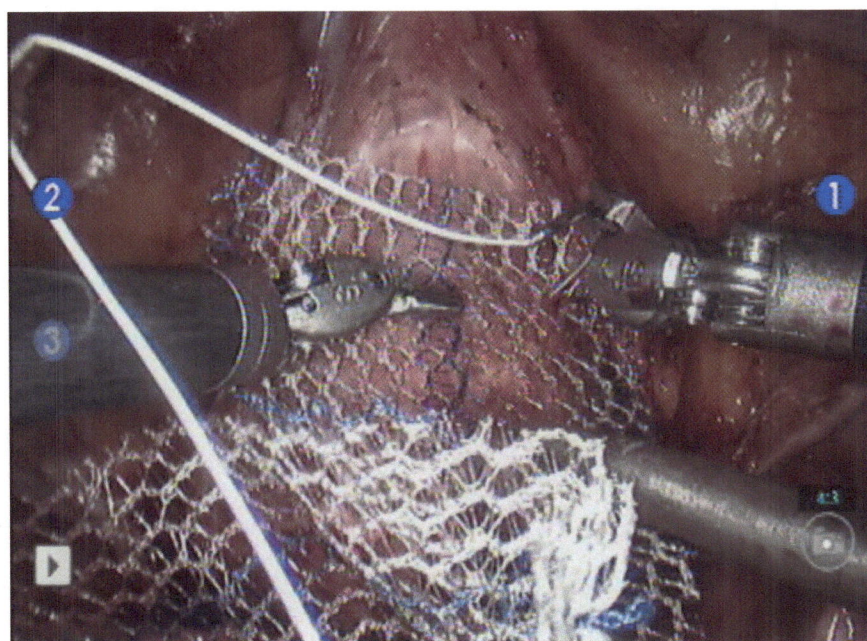

Figure 4: The y-shaped polypropylene mesh graft is first sutured to the anterior vaginal wall, starting at the distal corners. The bladder is retracted cephalad by the fourth arm.

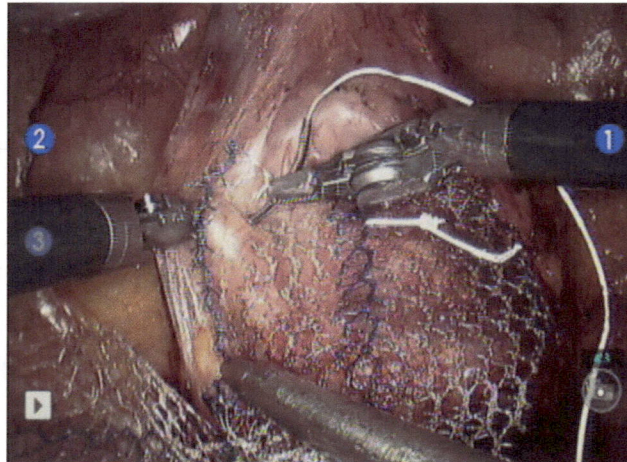

Figure 5: The y-shaped polypropylene mesh graft is first sutured to the anterior vaginal wall, starting at the distal corners. The bladder is retracted cephalad by the fourth arm.

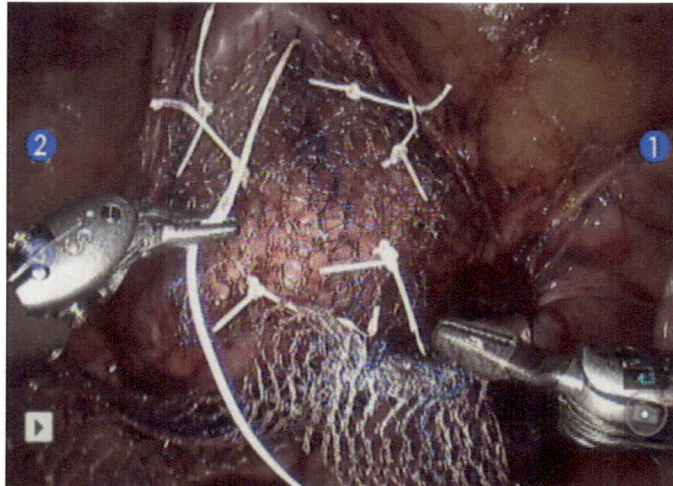

Figure 6: Completion of anterior mesh attachment using 6 sutures of 2-0 Gore-Tex®.

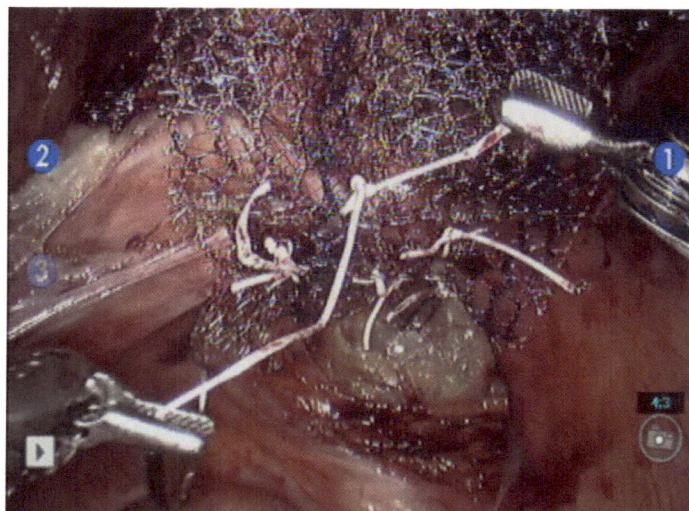

Figure 7: Attachment of posterior arm of mesh. Upward traction on the sacral portion of the mesh graft is provided by fourth arm.

The vagina is then deviated towards the sacrum, and the sacral arm of the mesh is pulled through the previously created retroperitoneal tunnel and, ensuring that no excessive tension exits, the sacral portion of the mesh graft is sutured to the anterior longitudinal ligament at the promontory using 2 or 3 interrupted sutures (Fig. **8**). When placing the needle during this critical juncture, it is important to rotate through the ligament along the curvature of the needle as opposed to driving the needle forward and potentially exiting further laterally than expected. Because of slight traction that exists on the mesh, a slip-knot is preferred over a surgeon's knot. Care is taken to visualize the middle sacral artery and either suture around, or cauterize it. If bleeding is encountered in this space, a ray-tec sponge can be introduced through the accessory port for manual compression. If bleeding continues, the use of floseal™ is recommended for controlling hemostasis.

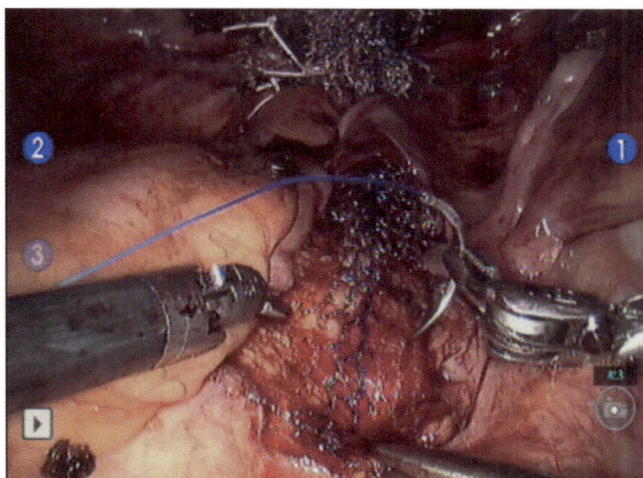

Figure 8: Mesh is directly sutured to the anterior longitudinal ligament using 2 or 3 stitches, secured with slip-knots. Care is taken to avoid undue tension on the mesh graft.

In an attempt to decrease the chance of postoperative bowel obstruction, the mesh is extraperitonealized using a 2-0 Vicryl™ suture cut to 10 inches. It is easiest to accomplish this task by starting at the vaginal apex with a purse-string like suture from the right anterior peritoneum to the right side of the cul-de-sac, coming over the mesh to pick up the left side of the incised peritoneum and then coming back through the left side of the bladder flap (Fig. **9**). A second stitch is then used to close the peritoneal window that was made at the sacral promontory.

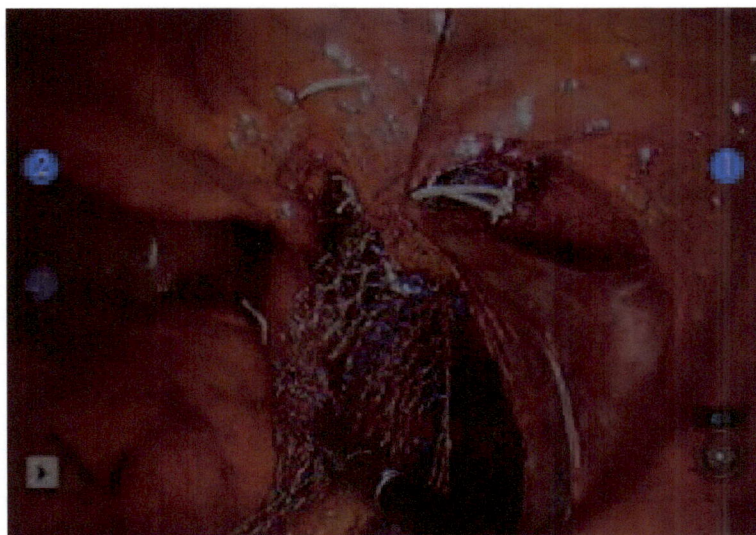

Figure 9: Mesh is extraperitonealized by closing the peritoneum from the apex of the vagina with a purse-string like stitch which is then continued to the promontory in a running fashion.

MODIFICATIONS FOR CERVICOSACROPEXY

In the event of an intact uterus and benign endometrial and cervical cytology, a supracervical hysterectomy is performed prior to the steps outlined above. Leaving the cervix in situ may reduce the chance of mesh erosion and it provides an excellent platform for mesh attachment. I find it most helpful to fully dissect the anterior and posterior vaginal walls prior to cervical amputation as the upward traction on the corpus improves visualization of the surgical planes. A useful and inexpensive instrument for vaginal manipulation when the cervix is present is the Colpo-Probe™ vaginal fornix delineator (Apple Medical, Marlborough MA) (Fig. **10**) that not only assists in dissection of the vagina from the bladder and rectum but also provides a stable surface during mesh attachment.

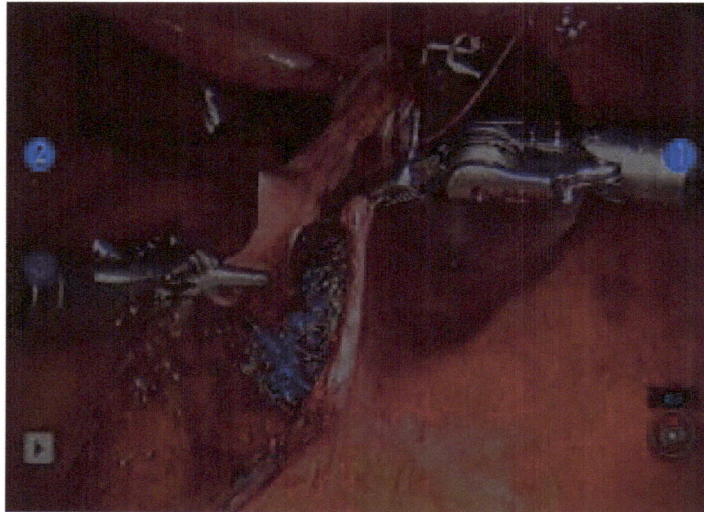

Figure 10: Mesh is extraperitonealized by closing the peritoneum from the apex of the vagina with a purse-string like stitch which is then continued to the promontory in a running fashion.

RESULTS

The studies that have evaluated the success of the robotic-assisted SCP have been limited in sample size and mean time of follow-up. A retrospective cohort study comparing short-term outcomes of RSCP to ASCP revealed a slight improvement in apical support at 6 weeks postoperatively, less blood loss, and a shorter hospital stay but was compromised by a significantly longer mean total operative time of 328 compared to 225 minutes. Rates of visceral injury were limited to one cystotomy in each group. Given the short duration of postoperative follow-up, an evaluation of mesh erosion was not possible [15]. A second retrospective cohort study of peri-operative outcomes of 80 women undergoing RSCP reported a mean operative time of 197 minutes, a 2.5% rate of bladder injury, 5% conversion to laparotomy, and 6% mesh erosion rate. Three patients (4%) developed recurrent POP within 6 months post surgery that required repeat operations [16]. Finally, one small retrospective case series of 30 patients who underwent RSCP with a mean follow up of 23 months reported a 3% conversion rate to laparotomy, 6.6% re-operation rate within 1 year, and 6.6% mesh erosion rate [17].

Surgical times using the robotic system may initially be longer but after completion of the learning curve, efficiency can be achieved. A retrospective review of 85 cases at VCU medical center reported a mean total surgical time of 194 ± 54 minutes [18]. which is substantially shorter than other published series.

CONCLUSION

The da Vinci™ surgical system facilitates completion of a colpo or cervicosacropexy in an identical manner to which it is performed in an open technique by surgeons who may not possess advanced laparoscopic skills. Full knowledge of the relevant anatomy is critical as significant morbidity can be encountered during the operation if incorrect surgical planes are created. We recommend proficiency with the open procedure before considering the robotic approach. Key points that must be considered during the procedure include the availability of a skilled bedside assistant who can direct a second assistant performing vaginal and rectal manipulation, use of steep trendelenburg position to remove the bowels from the operative field, correct identification of the sacral promontory, creation of a retroperitoneal tunnel, adequate dissection of the vesicovaginal and rectovaginal spaces, and individually fashioned y-shaped grafts. Adequate spacing between the robotic arms is essential to avoiding interference between instruments during the procedure therefore attention to port placement and docking is integral to the success of this procedure.

DISCLOSURE

Part of information included in this chapter has been previously published in "JOURNAL OF ROBOTIC SURGERY Volume 3, Number 1, 35-39.

REFERENCES

[1]   Nygaard I, Barber MD, Burgio KL, *et al.* Prevalence of symptomatic pelvic floor disorders in US women. JAMA. 2008; 300(11): 1311-1316.

[2]   Wu JM, Hundley AF, Fulton RG, Myers ER. Forecasting the prevalence of pelvic floor disorders in U.S. Women: 2010 to 2050. Obstet Gynecol. 2009; 114(6): 1278-1283.

[3]   Rooney K, Kenton K, Mueller ER, FitzGerald MP, Brubaker L. Advanced anterior vaginal wall prolapse is highly correlated with apical prolapse. Am J Obstet Gynecol. 2006; 195(6): 1837-1840.

[4]   Lowder JL, Park AJ, Ellison R, *et al.* The role of apical vaginal support in the appearance of anterior and posterior vaginal prolapse. Obstet Gynecol. 2008; 111(1): 152-157.

[5]   Summers A, Winkel LA, Hussain HK, DeLancey JO. The relationship between anterior and apical compartment support. Am J Obstet Gynecol. 2006; 194(5): 1438-1443.

[6]   Diwadkar GB, Barber MD, Feiner B, Maher C, Jelovsek JE. Complication and reoperation rates after apical vaginal prolapse surgical repair: a systematic review. Obstet Gynecol. 2009; 113(2 Pt 1): 367-373.

[7]   Nygaard IE, McCreery R, Brubaker L, *et al.* Abdominal sacrocolpopexy: a comprehensive review. Obstet Gynecol. 2004; 104(4): 805-823.

[8]   Maher C, Feiner B, Baessler K, Adams EJ, Hagen S, Glazener CM. Surgical management of pelvic organ prolapse in women. Cochrane Database Syst Rev. 2010; 4: CD004014.

[9]   Nezhat CH, Nezhat F, Nezhat C. Laparoscopic sacral colpopexy for vaginal vault prolapse. Obstet Gynecol. 1994; 84(5): 885-888.

[10]   Ross JW. Techniques of laparoscopic repair of total vault eversion after hysterectomy. J Am Assoc Gynecol Laparosc. 1997; 4(2): 173-183.

[11]   Cosson M, Rajabally R, Bogaert E, Querleu D, Crepin G. Laparoscopic sacrocolpopexy, hysterectomy, and burch colposuspension: feasibility and short-term complications of 77 procedures. JSLS. 2002; 6(2): 115-119.

[12]   Guenaga KK, Matos D, Wille-Jorgensen P. Mechanical bowel preparation for elective colorectal surgery. Cochrane Database Syst Rev. 2009; (1): CD001544.

[13]   Shveiky D, Aseff JN, Iglesia CB. Brachial plexus injury after laparoscopic and robotic surgery. J Minim Invasive Gynecol. 2010; 17(4): 414-420.

[14]   Matthews CA, Schubert CM, Woodward AP, Gill EJ. Variance in abdominal wall anatomy and port placement in women undergoing robotic gynecologic surgery. J Minim Invasive Gynecol. 2010; 17(5): 583-6.

[15]   Geller EJ, Siddiqui NY, Wu JM, Visco AG. Short-term outcomes of robotic sacrocolpopexy compared with abdominal sacrocolpopexy. Obstet Gynecol. 2008; 112(6): 1201-1206.

[16]   Akl MN, Long JB, Giles DL, *et al.* Robotic-assisted sacrocolpopexy: technique and learning curve. Surg Endosc. 2009; 23(10): 2390-2394.

[17]   Elliott DS, Krambeck AE, Chow GK. Long-term results of robotic assisted laparoscopic sacrocolpopexy for the treatment of high grade vaginal vault prolapse. J Urol. 2006; 176(2): 655-659.

[18]   Woodward A MC, Lamb E, Ramakrishnan V, Gill EJ.. Evaluation of surgical time, complications, and learning curve for robotic sacropexy. JMIG. 2010; 17(6): 32S.

CHAPTER 3

Robot-Assisted Myomectomy

Ceana Nezhat* and Shabnam Dadgar

Fellowship & Clinical Director, Nezhat Medical Center, Center for Special Minimally Invasive Surgery & Reproductive Medicine, Adjunct Clinical Associate Professor of Obstetrics & Gynecology, Stanford University School of Medicine, 5555 Peachtree Dunwoody Rd., Suite 276, Atlanta

Abstract: The use of robotics, or computer enhanced technology in laparoscopic myomectomy facilitates suturing and uterine reconstruction similar to laparotomy and LAM. It provides a 3-D view, eliminates tremor by downscaling movements, and superior range of motion. This makes laparoscopic suturing more intuitive in contrast to the counter-intuitive environment of LM, allowing proper reconstruction of uterine wall defects and minimizing risk of complications.

INTRODUCTION

Uterine myomas or fibroids are benign tumors of muscle cell origin. In the pelvis, most are found in the corpus of the uterus. Occasionally, myomas may be found in the fallopian tubes or the round ligaments and about 5% of uterine myomas originate from the cervix. Myomas are the most common uterine neoplasm, affecting 20 to 25% of women of reproductive age. They vary in size from microscopic to multinodular uterine tumors that can fill the patient's abdomen entirely.

SYMPTOMS

The severity and type of symptoms associated with uterine leiomyomas are dependent on their number, size and location. The most common symptoms are pressure from an enlarging pelvic mass, pain including dysmenorrhea and abnormal uterine bleeding. However, most women with uterine myomas are asymptomatic. An enlarged myoma or myomas often produce pressure symptoms similar to those of an enlarging pregnant uterus. Sometimes, an anterior myoma pressing on the bladder may produce urinary frequency and urgency. Very large myomas and broad ligament myomas may produce a unilateral or bilateral hydroureter. At times, myomas are the only identifiable abnormality after a detailed infertility investigation.

REPRODUCTIVE ISSUES IN WOMEN WITH FIBROIDS

The relationship between leiomyomas and infertility remains an ongoing subject of debate and the current data are conflicting. In this era of evidence-based medicine, additional randomized controlled studies of infertility patients with myomas are necessary to have clear results regarding the effect of fibroids in infertile patients [1]. In general, the incidence of myomas in infertile women without any obvious cause of infertility is 1-2.4 % [1]. Fibroids, especially those that press against the endometrium, may affect fertility by impairing implantation or causing abnormal uterine contractility.

The management of women with uterine fibroids depends on many factors including the size and location of the myoma, the patient's age and symptoms, the obstetrical history and future childbearing plans. The location of the fibroid(s) is a key factor in infertility and myomas that distort the uterine cavity increase the risk of miscarriage.

Most IVF centers prefer a patient who has a normal uterine cavity before proceeding with IVF. As a result, performing myomectomy in women planning to undergo IVF is a reasonable approach to increase her chances of a successful pregnancy. IVF success has decreased due to recent restrictions on the number of transferred embryos to

*Address correspondence to Ceana Nezhat: Fellowship & Clinical Director, Nezhat Medical Center, Center for Special Minimally Invasive Surgery & Reproductive Medicine, Adjunct Clinical Associate Professor of Obstetrics & Gynecology, Stanford University School of Medicine, 5555 Peachtree Dunwoody Rd., Suite 276, Atlanta, GA 30342, Tel: (404) 255-8778; Fax: (404) 255-5627; E-mail: ceana@nezhat.com

reduce the chances of multiple gestations. Therefore, with myomectomy and restoration of anatomy, not only does the chance of successful IVF increase, but the patient has a chance of spontaneous conception if no other limiting factors are present.

TREATMENT OF UTERINE LEIOMYOMAS

In general, asymptomatic uterine leiomyomas can be followed without intervention [2]. However, reassurance to women who are asymptomatic or have minimal symptoms is necessary, in order to avoid unnecessary intervention [3]. Prophylactic therapy is not advised except in women who are considering pregnancy with submucosal fibroids, and in those with moderate to severe hydronephrosis due to ureteral compression by fibroid [4]. In such instances, prophylactic myomectomy may enhance fertility and prevent miscarriage or urinary tract impairment.

Fibroids can be treated medically or surgically, depending on several factors such as the size, location, symptoms, fertility status and patient age [5]. Medical therapy is the first line of treatment when bleeding is the chief complaint.

Medical therapy provides adequate symptom relief in some women, primarily in situations where bleeding is the dominant or the only symptom. In general, 75% of women get some improvement over one year of therapy, but long-term failure rates are high [6]. Leiomyomas can be treated by techniques such as endometrial ablation, uterine artery embolization, magnetic resonance- guided focused- ultrasound surgery and myolysis. However, the most definitive treatment for a myomatous uterus is myomectomy. The indications for surgical therapy are persistent abnormal uterine bleeding, pain or pressure symptoms, rapidly enlarging pelvic mass, and treatment of infertility or recurrent pregnancy loss. Leiomyomas are the most common indication for hysterectomy, accounting for 30 percent of hysterectomies in whites and over 50% of hysterectomies in black women.

ROUTE OF MYOMECTOMY

The approach to myomectomy depends on the location of the myomas. Myomectomies can be done by laparotomy, vaginally, laparoscopically, hysteroscopically or robotically- assisted.

Hysteroscopic myomectomy is the procedure of choice for submucosal myomas [4,7] and vaginal myomectomy is the most appropriate technique for prolapsed myomas, Currently the conventional approach to myomectomy is open surgery, which is the standard practice in most places for women with intramural and multiple myomas, or when the uterus is significantly enlarged.

Abdominal myomectomy is performed through a large abdominal incision. After cutting and removing each uterine fibroid, the surgeon must carefully repair the uterine wall to minimize uterine bleeding, infection and scarring. However, as with any other abdominal surgery, adhesion formation, in particular adnexal adhesions, is worrisome in women of reproductive aged [8,9]. It is important to note that a vertical incision in the fundal area will avoid the cornua and as a result minimize the potential damage to the tubal ostia [10].

Advances in laparoscopic techniques such as suturing and instrumentation, have provided a minimally invasive alternative to laparotomy for subserosal, intramural and parasitic myomas. In experienced hands and with proper instrumentation, most myomectomies can be done laparoscopically. The laparoscopic approach is associated with faster recovery and potentially less adhesion formation, shorter hospital stay, decreased blood loss and a higher pregnancy rate [11-13]. Some studies have shown that pretreatment with GnRH agonists decreases blood loss and operating time, but this has not been shown in all studies [14].

Laparoscopic myomectomies (LM) are technically more challenging to perform, and there is also limited tactile sensation compared to abdominal myomectomies. Without proper suturing of the uterine defect, the risk of uterine rupture during subsequent pregnancy or during labor could be high. Studies have shown that there is a higher rate of complications in cases where fibroids are larger than 10 cm, and when more than 3 fibroids are removed [15,16]. Only surgeons who are trained to do laparoscopic suturing can perform laparoscopic myomectomy. However, this is an area of controversy as to whether reapproximation of the myometrium *via* laparoscopic suturing gives the uterine wall the same strength as multilayer closure at laparotomy [17].

Laparoscopically assisted myomectomy (LAM) is less difficult than LM and takes less time to perform, thereby making LAM a safe alternative to LM. LAM may be preferred over LM in cases with a myoma greater than 8 cm, multiple myomas requiring extensive morcellation, and/or deep, large, intramural myoma requiring uterine repair in multiple layers [18].

After mapping with standard laparoscopy and treating other pathology as need, the myomectomy is performed *via* a 3-4 cm mini-laparotomy. This allows for full palpation of the myometrium and also facilitates easier, faster, and more secure closure of the hysterotomy. Conventional uterine suturing in two or three layers reduces the potential for uterine dehiscence, fistulas, and adhesions. Morcellation is faster with diminished risk of seeding tissue. Postoperative pain and recovery are similar to LM [19].

Some of the major objectives of LAM are reduction of blood loss, prevention of postoperative adhesions, and maintenance of myometrial integrity. LAM, with "open" morcellation and conventional suturing, reduces the duration of the procedure and the need for more extensive laparoscopic experience.

ROBOTIC MYOMECTOMY

In spite of advancements in minimally invasive surgery, the majority of myomectomies are performed *via* laparotomy. This is believed to be due to technical limitations and lack of experience of surgeons with minimally invasive techniques [20]. Several studies in the literature have shown that robotics may facilitate the laparoscopic approach to myomectomy. (Table **1**) [17, 21-27].

In 2004, Advincula *et al.* described a retrospective case series of 35 patients who underwent robotic-assisted myomectomy. The mean number of myomas removed per patient was 1.6 (range 1-5) and the mean weight was 164.5 g. The majority of myomas were greater than 5 cm in size. The mean operating time was 230.8 minutes. The average estimated blood loss was 169 mL. In this study, three cases were converted to laparotomy, one due to cardiogenic shock from vasopressin injection (patient's history remarkable for Raynaud's disease), and the conversion of the other two cases was attributed to lack of tactile feedback. Postoperative complications included infection of the port site and aspiration pneumonia. The mean length of hospital stay was one day [21].

They also published additional data in 2007, where they compared surgical outcomes of myomectomy by robotic-assisted laparoscopy with those by conventional laparoscopy. They reported decreased estimated blood loss and complications rate, and the length of stay was significantly reduced in the robotic cohort (mean 1.5 days compared with 3.6 days). The rate of complications was higher in the laparotomy group and the cost of robotic-assisted myomectomy was higher compared to the conventional laparoscopy [17].

In 2006, Nezhat *et al.* published a case series of 15 patients who underwent a variety of gynecologic procedures. The procedures included treatment of endometriosis (6 cases), myomectomy (5 cases), total and supracervical hysterectomy (3 cases), ovarian cystectomy, sacral colpopexy (1 case), and Moschowitz procedure. The assembly time was 18.9 minutes (range 14 to 27), and the disassembly time was 2.1 minutes (range 1 to 3). There were no conversions to laparotomy [22].

In another study in 2009, Nezhat *et al.* compared robotic assisted myomectomy to conventional laparoscopic myomectomy in a retrospective matched control study. The groups were matched by age, body mass index, parity, previous abdominopelvic surgery, size, number and location of the myomas. The mean surgical time for the robotic myomectomy was 234 minutes (range 140–455) compared with 203 minutes (range 95–330) for laparoscopic myomectomy. Blood loss, length of stay, and postoperative complications were not significantly different [23].

Pitter *et al.* retrospectively reviewed 40 robot-assisted benign gynecological surgeries and concluded that there was a statistically significant decrease in the operative time for the cases performed later compared to the ones performed earlier. The mean estimated blood loss decreased as the number of the completed cases increased [25].

Mao *et al.* reported a case of a 38 year-old woman with a large uterine myoma (measuring approximately 9 x 8 x 7 cm, which was located at the anterior uterine wall). She underwent robotic -assisted myomectomy. The operative time was about 3 hours with an estimated blood loss of 150 mL [26].

Table 1

Study	# of patients	EBL (ml)	OR time (min)	Hospital stay (days)	# of Myomas	Weight of myomas (gr)	Intraoperative Complications	Postoperative Complications
Advincula [21] (2004)	35	169	230.8	1	1.6	164.5	Conversion to laparotomy (2) Cardiogenic shock (1)	Port site infection (1) Aspiration pneumonia (1)
Advincula [17] (2007) Robotic vs. LAP	29 vs. 29	195.69 vs. 364.66	231.8 vs.154.41	1.48 vs. 3.62	-	227.86 vs.223.76	Robotic: Cardiogenic shock (1) LAP: None	Robotic : Aspiration Pneumonia (1) port site cellulitis (1) Chest pain (1) LAP: Transfusion (2) Respiratory arrest (1) DVT (1) Acute renal failure (1) Hypertension (2) Fever (4) Hematoma (2) Wound dehiscence (1)
Nezhat [22] (2006)	15		Assembly: 18.9 Disassembly: 2.1				None	None
Nezhat [23] (2009) Robotic vs. LSC	15 vs. 35	370 vs. 420	234 vs. 203	1.00 vs. 1.05	3 vs. 4	116 vs. 156	None	None
Nezhat [24] (2009)	23		137				None	Bowel obstruction (1)
Pitter [23] (2008)	23	84.5	195.43		1-23	122.13	Additional ovarian cystectomy (1)	Bowel herniation (1)
Mao [26] (2007)	1	150	180	1	1		None	None
Bocca [27] (2007)	1			2 hours	1		None	None

Bocca *et al.* reported a 35-year-old woman who presented with secondary infertility, and a single 3 cm, predominantly intramural, fundal myoma. Robotic-assisted myomectomy was performed and following surgery, she conceived and delivered a healthy term infant by Caesarean section [27].

ROBOTIC VERSUS CONVENTIONAL LAPAROSCOPY

Even though conventional laparoscopy has had a major impact in gynecologic surgery, and the technology and equipment have advanced, it still has its own limitations including loss of haptics, loss of 3-dimensional (3-D) visualization, limited degree of motion and dexterity and amplification of physiologic tremors [20]. The innovation of robot-assisted laparoscopy has been a major break through in minimally invasive surgeries. Robot-assisted laparoscopy shares similar advantages over laparotomy with conventional laparoscopy, such as decreased morbidity and rapid recovery. In addition, it has unique features that help overcome the difficulties of conventional laparoscopy.

The major advantages of robot-assisted over conventional laparoscopy [28.29] are:

- Superior visualization — 3-D versus two-dimensional (2D) imaging of the operative field [20,24].
- Mechanical improvements — robotic instruments have seven degrees of freedom, similar to the human arm, wrist and hand, while conventional instruments have four degrees of freedom.

- Stabilization of instruments within the surgical field — in conventional laparoscopy, small movements by the surgeon are amplified (such as hand tremor) [20].

- Improved ergonomics for the operating surgeon — The surgeon can be seated with telerobotic systems [20,24,30,31]. which in turn results in less fatigue, and less pain and numbness in the arms, wrists, or shoulders after the surgery [32].

- Faster learning curve for suturing [24].

The study that Nezhat *et al.* conducted in 2006, concluded that robotic- assisted procedures have advantages in providing a 3-D visualization of the field, decreased fatigue and the tremor of the surgeon, as well as added wrist motion for improved dexterity. The established disadvantages in their study were cost, extra time needed for assembly and disassembly of the equipment and the bulkiness of the system [22].

Limitations of robotic surgery

The current limitations of robotic technology [28] include:

- Additional surgical training and time [20]
- Increased costs and operating theatre time
- Bulkiness of the devices [33]
- Increased operating time for assembly and disassembly [33]
- The initial expense of the robot [20]
- Instrumentation limitations (e.g., lack of a robotic suction and irrigation device, size, cost)
- Absence of tactile sensation [20]
- Risk of mechanical failure
- Limited number of energy sources, such as laser
- Not designed for abdominal surgery involving more than one quadrant
- Larger canula site compared to laparoscopy [20]
- New technology, unproven benefit [20]

It should be noted that robotic surgery is an evolving technology with constant improvement, and many of these limitations will likely resolve in time. Since the introduction of the *daVinci* System we have seen three generations of robots with significant improvement at each transition.

APPLICATIONS OF ROBOTIC SURGERY

Robotic surgery has been successfully applied in cardiac surgery [34], urology [35], general surgery [36], orthopedics [37], ophthalmology [38], neurosurgery [39], and gynecology [40-45] including gynecologic oncology [45,46].

Currently, a number of female pelvic ablative and reconstructive procedures are being performed with the use of the surgical robot including myomectomies, tubal reanastomosis, endometriosis, oophorectomies, ovarian cystectomies, and total and supracervical hysterectomies. In urogynecology it has been applied to sacralcolpopexy and uterovesical fistulas. In oncology, the robot has been adopted for radical hysterectomies in cervical cancer, pelvic and para-aortic lymphadenectomies, trachelectomies, as well as its utility in endometrial and ovarian cancer [20].

Nezhat *et al.* reported a successful case of robotic-assisted trachelectomy after supracervical hysterectomy in a 40 year old female with a history of severe endometriosis and adhesions, who presented with persistent pain and bleeding after abdominal supracervical hysterectomy. There was minimal blood loss and no intraoperative or postoperative complications reported [47].

A 2009 review of the literature about the application of robotics to gynecologic oncology revealed 38 articles, and 27 were included in the study. The data suggested that estimated blood loss, operative time, length of hospital stay and complications were comparable between robotic and laparoscopic surgery for gynecologic cancer. The robotic-assisted laparoscopic surgeries were associated with more lymphocysts, lymphoceles and lymphedema compared to laparoscopy and laparotomy in patients with cervical cancer. Infectious and lung-related morbidity, postoperative ileus and bleeding or clot formation were more commonly reported in the laparotomy group compared with the other 2 cohorts in patients with endometrial cancer. There is good evidence that robotic surgery facilitates laparoscopic surgery with comparable surgical outcome and operative time, shorter hospital stay and fewer complications than with surgeries done *via* laparotomy [48].

BASIC SET UP OF ROBOT

A surgical robotic system consists of three parts: a patient-side robot, a vision cart, and the robotic master console. The surgeon operates from the remote master console. The console operates with hand controls and foot pedals. One of the foot pedals controls the camera movement, and repositioning of hand controls is provided by another foot pedal. The third set of foot pedals controls monopolar and bipolar energy sources. The docking involves bringing the robot in between the patient's legs or at her side (side docking) and attaching the robotic arms to canulas.

EndoWrist® Instrumentation

A variety of *EndoWrist* instruments are available for use during a myomectomy. Instruments such as the bipolar PK™ dissecting forceps, hot shears (monopolar curved shears), and tenaculum and mega needle driver allow for safe completion of a myomectomy. Harmonic shears are available for use with the robot, however it lacks articulation at the tip.

Operating Room Set Up

Prior to transferring the patient into the operating room the scrub nurse prepares two instrument tables—one for abdominal and the other for vaginal manipulations, and the robotic arms are draped.

Positioning the Patient

Patient is under general endotracheal anesthesia, and in dorsal lithotomy position. The arms are padded and tucked at their sides using cushioned stirrups [40]. The proper use of shoulder braces or foam is important to avoid patient slippage during the Trendelenburg position. The patient is then placed in Trendelenburg positioning (30 to 45 degrees).

Examination under anesthesia is performed before the patient is prepped and draped. The bladder is drained with a Foley catheter, and a uterine manipulator, such as the HUMI (Cooper Surgical, Trumbull, CT), is placed in order to facilitate the robot-assisted myomectomy.

Port placement

Initial abdominal entry is done either by open technique, Veress needle, or direct insertion, depending on the surgeon's experience and preference [49]. Based on the recommendations of the manufacturer (Intuitive Surgical), the port for the scope and camera should be placed 10 to 20 cm away from the target organ. Two sizes of scopes are available, 12 mm and 8.5 mm. Illumination is stronger with the 12 mm scope and is preferable for wide view visualization. The 8.5 mm scope is preferable for supraumbilical ports with focused targets, which provides better visualization.

A 12 mm port is placed on the medial line at or above the umbilicus, depending on the size of the uterus. As a general rule, approximately 8–10 cm distance between the endoscope and the top of the uterus or leiomyoma during manipulation is essential during myomectomy, due to the enucleation process resulting in the fibroid moving out and toward the endoscope.

The remaining ports placements are as follows:

1. Port for the first robotic working arm— an 8 mm trocar is placed hands-breadth distance (8–12 cm) on the right and 15°–30° distally from the camera port.

2. Port for the second robotic working arm— an 8 mm trocar is placed hands-breadth distance (8–12 cm) on the left and 15°–30° distally from the camera port.

3. Port for the third robotic working arm— an 8 mm trocar, 8–12 cm laterally from the port for the second working arm.

4. Port 1 for assistance— 5 mm trocar, 8–12 cm laterally from the port for the first working arm.

5. Port 2 for assistance— 10 mm trocar, 8–10 cm distally from port 1 for assistance.

A dilute solution of vasopressin, 20 units in 60-100 mL of NaCl, is injected into the myometrium around the fibroid using a 7 inch 22-gauge spinal needle placed directly through the anterior abdominal wall. After adequate blanching of the myometrium around the myoma is obtained, an incision is made on the serosa covering the fibroid with a monopolar or harmonic device.

It is important that the incision is made in a longitudinal axis in order to facilitate the suturing process and to identify the appropriate plane. Once the plane is found, the myoma is enucleated using blunt dissection, creating traction and countertraction. Care should be taken to minimize use of energy on the myometrium to avoid delayed tissue necrosis. If additional exposure is needed, the fourth arm can be used for traction/countertraction on the myoma, or it can be done by the bedside assistant with a tenaculum.

After complete removal of the fibroid, the suturing process will take place by either interrupted sutures of 0-Vicryl on CT-2 needles cut to six inches, or running sutures of 0-Vicryl on CT-2 needles cut to 11 inches. Suture passage and exchange are managed through the accessory port by the bedside assistant. It is critical to repair the deep layers of the incision in multilayer fashion. Once the myometrial layer is closed, the serosa is sutured with a running baseball stitch of 3-0 Vicryl on a HS needle. Recently, we have been using barbed suture, Quill™ SRS (Angiotech Pharmaceuticals, Vancouver, BC, Canada) 7 inch length, double stranded with 2-0 and 3-0 strands for running layer closure of the muscularis and serosa with good results. At the time of closure of the uterine defect, if multiple leiomyomas are to be removed, it is better to repair each uterine defect separately [50,51].

The robotic device should then be undocked, and with the use of a morcellator that is placed through the accessory port, the extraction of leiomyomata from the abdomen will begin. There are different mechanical and electric morcellators available. We have had good experience with the Rotocut (Karl Storz Endoscopy, El Segundo, CA) morcellator. There are variable sized canula blades (12 and 15 mm) and has the highest speed (1200 RMP) available, providing versatility. Additionally, only the blade is disposable; therefore in cases of large and calcified myomas, when the blade dulls it is changed out for a new one and the rest of the morcellator remains. After morcellation, copious irrigation is necessary to remove all debris to minimize risk of parasitic myomas [52]. Once hemostasis is ensured and the abdomen irrigated, an adhesion barrier is placed over all uterine incisions [50,51]. All instruments are then removed from the patient's abdomen and pneumoperitoneum released. Port sites are closed accordingly.

REFERENCES

[1] Donnez J, Jadoul P. What are the implications of myomas on fertility? A need for a debate? Hum Reprod 2002; 17: 1424-30

[2] Parker WH. Uterine myomas: management. Fertil Steril 2007; 88: 255-71.

[3] Carlson KJ, Miller BA, Fowler FJ Jr. The Maine Women's Health Study: I. Outcomes of hysterectomy. Obstet Gynecol 1994; 83: 556-65

[4] Lefebvre G, Vilos G, Allaire C, Jeffrey J, Arneja J, Birch C, Fortier M, Wagner MS. The management of uterine leiomyomas. J Obstet Gynaecol Can 2003; 25: 396-418

[5] Stewart EA. Uterine fibroids. Lancet 2001; 27: 293-8

[6] Carlson KJ, Miller BA, Fowler FJ Jr. The Maine Women's Health Study: II. Outcomes of nonsurgical management of leiomyomas, abnormal bleeding, and chronic pelvic pain. Obstet Gynecol 1994; 83: 566-72

[7] Ubaldi F, Tournaye H, Camus M, Van der Pas H, Gepts E, Devroey P. Fertility after hysteroscopic myomectomy. Hum Reprod Update 1995; 1: 81-90

[8] Tulandi T, Murray C, Guralnick M. Adhesion formation and reproductive outcome after myomectomy and second-look laparoscopy. Obstet Gynecol 1993; 82: 213-5

[9]   Fauconnier A, Dubuisson JB, Ancel PY, Chapron C. Prognostic factors of reproductive outcome after myomectomy in infertile patients. Hum Reprod 2000; 15: 1751-7

[10]   Guarnaccia MM, Rein MS. Traditional surgical approaches to uterine fibroids: abdominal myomectomy and hysterectomy. Clin Obstet Gynecol 2001; 44: 385-400

[11]   Bulletti C, Polli V, Negrini V, Giacomucci E, Flamigni C. Adhesion formation after laparoscopic myomectomy. J Am Assoc Gynecol Laparosc 1996; 3: 533-6

[12]   Seracchioli R, Rossi S, Govoni F, Rossi E, Venturoli S, Bulletti C, Flamigni C. Fertility and obstetric outcome after laparoscopic myomectomy of large myomata: a randomized comparison with abdominal myomectomy. Hum Reprod 2000; 15: 2663-8

[13]   Palomba S, Zupi E, Falbo A, Russo T, Marconi D, Tolino A, Manguso F, Mattei A, Zullo F. A multicenter randomized, controlled study comparing laparoscopic versus minilaparotomic myomectomy: reproductive outcomes. Fertil Steril 2007; 88: 933-41.

[14]   Campo S, Garcea N. Laparoscopic myomectomy in premenopausal women with and without preoperative treatment using gonadotrophin-releasing hormone analogues. Hum Reprod 1999; 14: 44-8

[15]   Sizzi O, Rossetti A, Malzoni M, Minelli L, La Grotta F, Soranna L, Panunzi S, Spagnolo R, Imperato F, Landi S, Fiaccamento A, Stola E. Italian multicenter study on complications of laparoscopic myomectomy. Minim Invasive Gynecol 2007; 14: 453-62

[16]   Hanafi M. Predictors of leiomyoma recurrence after myomectomy. Obstet Gynecol 2005; 105: 877-81

[17]   Advincula AP, Xu X, Goudeau S 4th, Ransom SB. Robot-assisted laparoscopic myomectomy versus abdominal myomectomy: a comparison of short-term surgical outcomes and immediate costs. J Minim Invasive Gynecol 2007; 14: 698–705

[18]   Nezhat C, Nezhat F, Bess O, Nezhat CH, Mashiach R. Laparoscopically assisted myomectomy: a report of a new technique in 57 cases. Int J Fertil 1994; 39: 39-44

[19]   Glasser M. Minimally invasive approaches to myomectomy. In: Nezhat C, Nezhat F, Nezhat CH, eds. Nezhat's Operative Gynecologic Laparoscopy and Hysteroscopy. 3rd edition. New York: Cambridge University Press, 2008; 40-56

[20]   Cho JE, Shamshirsaz AH, Nezhat CH, Nezhat C, Nezhat F. New technology for reproductive medicine: laparoscopy, endoscopy, robotic surgery and gynecology: a review of the literature. Minerva Gynecol 2009; 61

[21]   Advincula AP, Song A, Burke W, Reynolds RK. Preliminary experience with robotic-assisted laparoscopic myomectomy. J Am Assoc Gynecol Laparosc 2004; 11: 511-8

[22]   Nezhat C, Saberi NS, Shahmohamady B, Nezhat F. Robotic-assisted laparoscopy in gynecological surgery. J Soc Laparosc Surg 2006; 10: 317-20

[23]   Nezhat C, Lavie O, Hsu S, Watson J, Barnett O, Lemyre M. Robotic-assisted laparoscopic myomectomy compared with standard laparoscopic myomectomy – a retrospective matched control study. Fertil 2009; 91: 556-9

[24]   Nezhat C, Lavie O, Lemyre M, Unal E, Nezhat CH, Nezhat F. Robotic-assisted laparoscopic surgery. Scientific dream or reality? Fertil Steril 2009; 91: 2620-2

[25]   Pitter MC, Anderson P, Blisset A, Pemberton N. Robotic-assisted gynecological surgery-establishing training criteria minimizing operating time and blood loss. Int J Med Robot 2008; 4: 114-20

[26]   Mao SP, Lai HC, Chang FW, Yu MH, Chang CC. Laparoscopy- assisted robotic myomectomy using the daVinci system. Taiwan J Obstet Gynecol 2007; 46: 174-6

[27]   Bocca S, Stadtmauer L, Oehninger S. Uncomplicated full term pregnancy after da Vinci- assisted laparoscopic myomectomy. Repo Biomed Online 2007; 14: 246-9

[28]   Bhayani SB. Laparoscopic partial nephrectomy: fifty cases. Endourol 2008; 22: 313-6

[29]   Oppenheimer P, Weghorst S, MacFarlane M, Sinanan M. Immersive surgical robotic interfaces. Stud Health Technol Inform 1999; 62: 242-8

[30]   Stylopoulos N, Rattner D. Robotics and ergonomics. Surg Clin North Am 2003; 83: 1321-37

[31]   Sroga J, Patel SD, Falcone T. Robotics in reproductive medicine. Front Biosci 2008; 1: 1308-17

[32]   Berguer R, Forkey DL, Smith WD. Ergonomic problems associated with laparoscopic surgery. Surg Endosc 1999; 13: 466-8

[33]   Nezhat C, Lavie O, Lemyre M, Gemer O, Bhagan L, Nezhat CH. Laparoscopic hysterectomy with and without a robot: Stanford experience. JSLS 2009; 13: 125-128

[34]   Boehm DH, Reichenspurner H, Gulbins H, *et al.* Early experience with robotic technology for coronary artery surgery. Ann Thorac Surg 1999; 68: 1542–1546

[35]   Binder J, Brautigam R, Jonas D, Bentas W. Robotic surgery in urology: fact or fantasy? BJU Int 2004; 94: 1183–1187

[36]   Melvin WS, Needleman BJ, Krause KR, *et al.* Computer enhanced robotic telesurgery. Initial experience in foregut surgery. Surg Endosc 2002; 16: 1790 –1792

[37] Bargar WL. Robots in orthopaedic surgery: past, present, and future. Clin Orthop 1998; 354: 82–91

[38] Yu DY, Cringle SJ, Constable IJ. Robotic ocular ultramicrosurgery. Aust N Z J Ophthalmol 1998; 26: S6 –S8

[39] Spetzger U, Gilsbach JM, Mosges R, Schlondorff G, Laborde G. The computer-assisted localizer, a navigational help in microneurosurgery. Eur Surg Res 1997; 29 : 481– 487

[40] Nezhat C, Lavie O, Hsu S, Watson J, Barnett O, Lemyre M. Robotic-assisted laparoscopic myomectomy compared with standard laparoscopic myomectomy-a retrospective matched control study. Fertil Steril 2009; 91: 556 –559

[41] Falcone T, Goldberg JM, Margossian H, Stevens L. Robotic assisted laparoscopic microsurgical tubal anastomosis: a human pilot study. Fertil Steril 2000; 73: 1040 –1042

[42] Falcone T, Steiner CP. Robotically assisted gynaecological surgery. Hum Fertil 2002; 5: 72–74

[43] Falcone T, Goldberg JM. Robotics in gynecology. Surg Clin North Am 2003; 83: 1483–1489

[44] Nezhat C, Saberi NS, Shahmohamady B, Nezhat F. Robotic assisted laparoscopy in gynecological surgery. JSLS 2006; 10: 317–320

[45] Nezhat FR, Datta MS, Liu C, Chuang L, Zakashansky K. Robotic radical hysterectomy versus total laparoscopic radical hysterectomy with pelvic lymphadenectomy for treatment of early cervical cancer. JSLS 2008; 12: 227–237

[46] Field JB, Benoit MF, Dinh TA, az-Arrastia C. Computer enhanced robotic surgery in gynecologic oncology. Surg Endosc 2007; 21: 244 –246

[47] Nezhat CH, Rogers JD. Robot-assisted laparoscopic trachelectomy after supracervical hysterectomy. Fertil Steril 2008; 90: 850.e1–e3

[48] Cho JE, Nezhat FR, Robotics and gynecologic oncology: review of the literature. J Minim Invas Gynecol 2009; 16: 669–681

[49] Nezhat C, Nezhat CH, Nezhat F, Ferland R. Laparoscopic Access: principles of laparoscopy. In: Nezhat C, Nezhat F, Nezhat CH, eds. Nezhat's Operative Gynecologic Laparoscopy and Hysteroscopy. 3rd edition. New York: Cambridge University Press, 2008; 40-56

[50] Mettler L, Audebert A, Lehmann-Willenbrock E, Schive-Peterhansl, K, Jacobs VR. Adhesion barrier system in patients undergoing myomectomy. Fertil Steril 2004; 82: 398–404

[51] Pellicano M, Bramante S, Cirillo D, Palomba S, Bifulco G, Zullo,F, Nappi C. Effectiveness of autocrosslinked hyaluronic acid gel after laparoscopic myomectomy in infertile patients. Fertil Steril 2003; 80: 441–444

[52] Kho K, Nezhat CH. Parasitic Myomas. Obstet Gynecol 2009; 114: 611-5

CHAPTER 4

Robotic Assisted Laparoscopic Hysterectomy

Michael C. Pitter

Department of Obstetrics & Gynecology, Newark Beth Israel Medical Center, Newark, Newark, New Jersey USA

Abstract: Hysterectomy is the most common major gynecologic surgery performed in the United States, second only to cesarean section. Over 500,000 of these procedures are performed each year using a variety of treatment modalities. The abdominal approach is by far the most common comprising of up to 64%. Laparoscopic hysterectomies make up only 14 % [1]. When one examines the different approaches to hysterectomy in the United States, the number of vaginal hysterectomies over the past 10 years has not changed significantly.

In April 2005, the FDA approved the use of the da Vinci Surgical System™ for surgery in Gynecology. This provided another option for surgeons other than the previously described methods. Recent data shows that the number of hysterectomies performed by the laparoscopic technique has the potential to increase by using computer enhanced telemanipulation otherwise known as Robotic Surgery [2].

Key Words: da Vinci surgery, robotic hysterectomy, fibroid uterus.

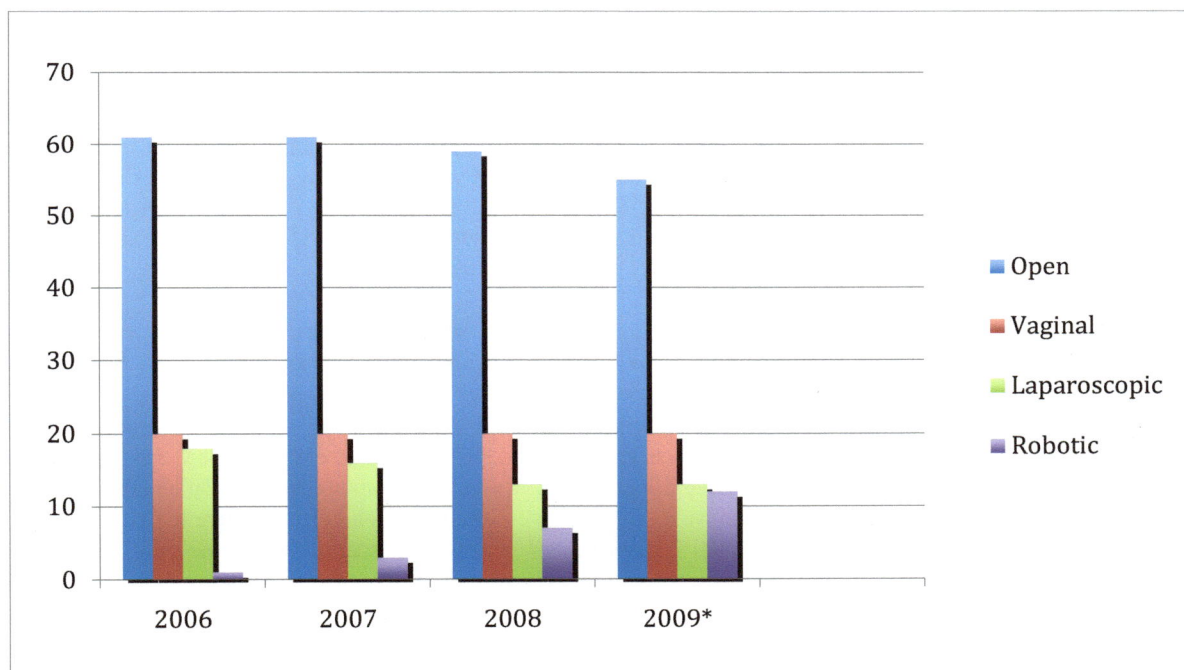

Hysterectomy in the United States (Projected trend; Source: Solucient Data).

DEFINITIONS

- Laparoscopic Assisted Vaginal Hysterectomy (LAVH) – Vaginal hysterectomy facilitated by laparoscopy, including removal of the adnexa, lysis of adhesions but not ligation of the uterine vessels.

- Laparoscopic Subtotal or Supracervical Hysterectomy (LSH or LASH) – Removal of the fundus of the uterus above the level of the upper cervix but below the uterine vessels with laparoscopic assistance. The cervix is left in situ.

*Address correspondence to Michael C. Pitter: Chief of Gynecological Robotic & Minimally Invasive Surgery, Newark Beth Israel Medical Center, 201 Lyons Avenue, Newark, New Jersey USA 07112; Tel: 973-926-4600; E-mail: mail@drpitter.net

- Total Laparoscopic Hysterectomy (TLH) – Removal of the uterus and cervix with complete detachment of the cardinal-uterosacral ligament complex with repair of the vagina via laparoscopic guidance.

- Robotic Assisted Laparoscopic Hysterectomy – Use of the surgical robot to assist the conduct of laparoscopic hysterectomy. It could be total or subtotal hysterectomy.

SEARCH STRATEGY AND STUDY SELECTION

During an interval of six years, the number of publications on robotic surgery and in particular, robotic hysterectomy has increased exponentially. A search was performed with the English language as a filter using the following bibliographic databases: Cochrane Database of Systematic Reviews, PubMed-Medline. The search words included robotic hysterectomy, da Vinci hysterectomy and robotic assisted laparoscopic hysterectomy. The results showed that there was a paucity of randomized controlled studies. A total of 20 published articles were included for data analysis.

HISTORY

In 1989, Reich [3] published a report of the first laparoscopic hysterectomy. Prior to this, the two techniques of hysterectomy included open abdominal and vaginal hysterectomy. His novel approach transformed the use of the laparoscope from merely a diagnostic tool to a more prominent position in the minimally invasive surgical armamentarium. The idea was to convert an abdominal hysterectomy into either vaginal hysterectomy or total laparoscopic hysterectomy especially in the case of extensive adhesive disease such as endometriosis or multiple prior laparotomy procedures.

At that time circa 1990, laparoscopic hysterectomy made up only 0.3% of all hysterectomies performed in the United States [4]. Since then technology has advanced significantly especially in the area of video CCD (controlled coupling devices) and illumination sources for use in endoscopy. Digital high definition quality images have replaced the shadowy pictures of the early 1990's. In addition, an array of instruments has replaced the Kleppinger bipolar forceps formerly a mainstay for vessel sealing. Computers and the concept of surgical robotics were almost simultaneously introduced starting with the work of the National Aeronautics and Space Administration (NASA) and the Defense Advanced Research Projects Agency (DARPA).

An Automated Endoscopic System for Optimal Positioning (AESOP) was first developed to give the surgeon more control over complicated operations by freeing up one surgeon's hand from holding the laparoscope. This enabled two or more surgeons to tackle more complicated operations laparoscopically. The system was subsequently proved to be problematic and unreliable. Schurr *et al.* [5] in May 2000 described a master-slave manipulator system known as Advanced Robotic Telemanipulator for Minimally Invasive Surgery (ARTEMIS). This early robotic technology provided the surgeon with increased degrees of freedom. Both the Zeus robotic system (Computer Motion, Goleta, CA) and the da Vinci robotic system (Intuitive Surgical, Sunnyvale, CA) evolved from this platform of remote telemanipulators. Computer Motion and its products were eventually absorbed by Intuitive Surgical. To date, the only commercially available telerobotic system available for use in minimally invasive surgery is the da Vinci Surgical System.

SURGICAL SYSTEM AND RELATED EQUIPMENT

The da Vinci Surgical System consists of a surgical console, a patient cart and a vision tower (Fig. **1**). There are currently three generations of this system available worldwide. The "Standard" is commonly regarded as the first generation system. The "S" system comes with two variations the "S" and "S" HD and finally the "Si". The distinguishing characteristics between the "Standard" and the "S" systems are the longer instruments on the "S" in addition to greater range or motion and pitch. The "S" systems also come with three instrument arms and a camera arm with all machines.

The HD system on the "S HD" provides a High Definition 3 D view of the operative field with the ability to obtain a panoramic aspect ratio of 16:9 that is 30 % wider with 20 % more viewing area. It also has a digital zoom reducing interference between the endoscope and the instruments. The "Si" system improved on the "S" by integrating some of the components from the surgeon's console into the vision cart and providing more options on the use of energy sources in addition to improving the visual experience.

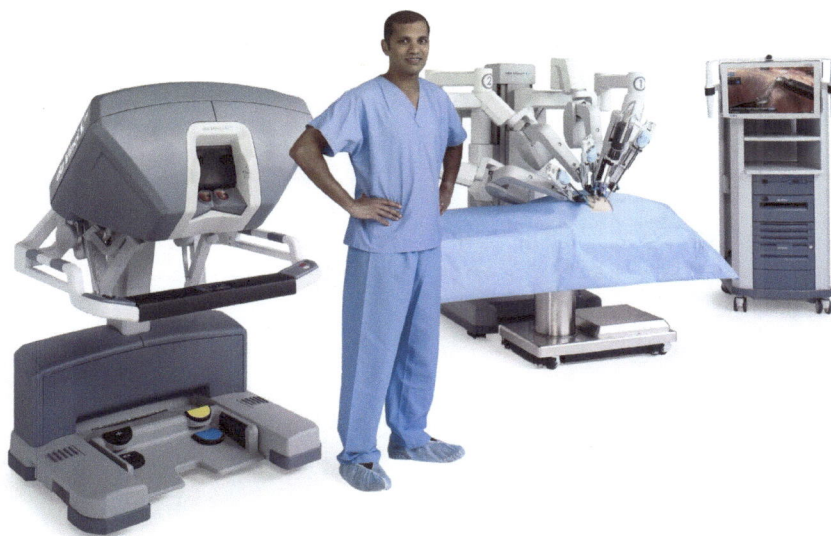

Figure 1: From left to right – Surgeon's Console, Patient Cart and Vision Tower. Courtesy of Intuitive Surgical Inc., Sunnyvale, California USA.

The surgeon sits at the console several meters away from the patient and is able to view the operation using the stereoscopic 3D, High Definition binoculars. There are three sizes of endoscopes available; 12 mm, 8.5 mm and a 5 mm. The 5 mm endoscope is the only one that does not provide a 3 D image. In addition to the camera and endoscope, there are three instruments that may be used to perform the operations with the surgeon having control over two at a given time.

There are two sizes of instruments available. The standard size is the 8 mm, while the 5 mm size is typically not used for hysterectomy. The instruments are tiny and EndoWristed® to provide the surgeon with 7 degrees of motion with tremor reduction and motion scaling. This allows the surgeon to perform precise and complicated procedures within the confines of the pelvis during laparoscopy. These instruments eliminate the fulcrum effect seen in conventional laparoscopy [6]. They are controlled using master controllers and foot pedals as previously described [5].

There are several instruments that may be used to perform the hysterectomy. The author is a strong proponent of using all three instrument arms during the hysterectomy. Others use two instruments arms only [*]. Instrumentation should include a grasper such as a Prograsp™ or a Cadiére™, HotShears™ or similar device to deliver monopolar cutting energy *i.e.*, Hook or Spatula and a bipolar device. The types of bipolar devices used vary depending on the surgeon's preference.

The devices available are the Precise™, Fenestrated™ and Maryland™ bipolar instruments and the PK Dissector™ (Gyrus ACMI, Maplegrove, MN). The PK Dissector is the only non-fenestrated advanced bipolar device and has an impedance monitor to alert the surgeon when complete tissue desiccation has been achieved. At the completion of the hysterectomy needle drivers are used to place sutures when applicable.

TECHNIQUE

Benign conditions account for 90% of all hysterectomies [7]. The objective of this chapter is on robotic hysterectomy for non-malignant indications such as symptomatic leiomyomata uteri, dysfunctional uterine bleeding, endometriosis, or adenomyosis. The American Association of Gynecological Laparoscopists (AAGL) classification for laparoscopic hysterectomy is used to describe the surgical approach [8]. The commonly used techniques are AAGL Type IVE (total laparoscopic removal of the uterine corpus and cervix including vaginal cuff closure) and LSH III (Table **1**).

Table 1: AAGL Classification of Laparoscopic Hysterectomy

Type	Description
Type 0	Laparoscopic---directed preparation for vaginal hysterectomy
Type 1	Dissection up to but not including uterine arteries *Type IA* Ovarian artery pedicle(s) only *Type IB1* I A + anterior structures *Type IC* I A + posterior culdotomy *Type ID1* I A + anterior structures and posterior culdotomy
Type II	Type I + uterine artery occlusion and division, unilateral or bilateral *Type IIA* Ovarian artery(ies) and uterine artery(ies) occlusion and division only *Type IIB1* II A + anterior structures *Type IIC* II A + posterior culdotomy *Type IID1* II A + anterior structures and posterior culdotomy
Type III	*Type II* + portion of cardinal-uterosacral ligament complex only, unilateral or bilateral *Type IIIA* Uterine and ovarian artery pedicles with portion of the cardinal-uterosacral complex only, unilateral or bilateral *Type IIIB1* III A + anterior structures *Type IIIC* III A + posterior culdotomy *Type IIID1* III A + anterior structures and posterior culdotomy
Type IV	*Type II* + total cardinal-uterosacral ligament complex, unilateral or bilateral *Type IVA* Uterine and ovarian artery pedicles with complete detachment of the total cardinal-uterosacral ligament complex only, unilateral or bilateral *Type IVB1 IV A + anterior structures* *Type IVC IV A + posterior culdotomy* *Type IVD1 IV A + anterior structures and posterior culdotomy* *Type IVE Laparoscopically directed removal of entire uterus*

The system describes the portion of the procedure completed laparoscopically. * A suffix "o" may be added if unilateral or bilateral oophorectomy is performed 1 - The B and D subgroups may be further subclassified according to the degree of dissection involving the bladder and whether an anterior culdotomy is created: Reference - Journal of Obstetrics and Gynecology, Vol. 82(4), pp 625).

Cadiére *et al.* [9] in 2001 described the first robotic assisted laparoscopic hysterectomy. The year after, Diaz-Arrastia *et al.* [10] published a report on the first series of hysterectomy with robotic assistance. The operative times ranged from 4.5 to 10 hours and the estimated blood loss (EBL) from 50 to 1500 ml. Reynolds *et al.* described a larger series of 16 patients with a mean operative time of 242 minutes (170–432) and mean hospital stay of 1.5 days [6]. Robotic hysterectomy for complicated cases involving patients with scarred or obliterated anterior cul-de-sac was described by Advincula *et al.* [11].

Basic Set-Up

The patient is placed in a low lithotomy position after induction of general endotracheal anesthesia. Both arms are tucked and placed by the side and the breasts and faced padded for protection. Caution must be used to avoid hyperextending the elbows and externally rotating the arms to prevent ulnar nerve injury. Given the range of motion of the instruments and camera arms, the forearms, breasts and face should be protected from the arm excursions with padding (Fig. **2**). During the tucking process, the patient can either be placed on a gel pad or on a deflatable bean bag. This is to prevent skidding or slipping on the operating room table in steep Trendelenburg position. Shoulder braces may increase risk of brachial nerve injury and should be avoided.

After the patient is prepped and draped, an indwelling catheter is placed inside the bladder and a uterine manipulator is inserted. There are a number of uterine manipulators available that provide a means for distinguishing the cervico-vaginal junction required for the laparoscopic colpotomy incision. A method of establishing pneumo-occlusion is also important. The two types of manipulators commonly used are the VCare® system (ConMed Endosurgery, Utica, NY, USA) and the RUMI™Uterine Manipulator (Cooper Surgical, Trumball, CT, USA). There are other systems notably the McCartney tube (Tyco HealthCare, Inc., Sydney, Australia) that is comprised of a disposable silicone tube with one end in the vaginal fornices and the other outside the vagina and capped to maintain pneumo-occlusion.

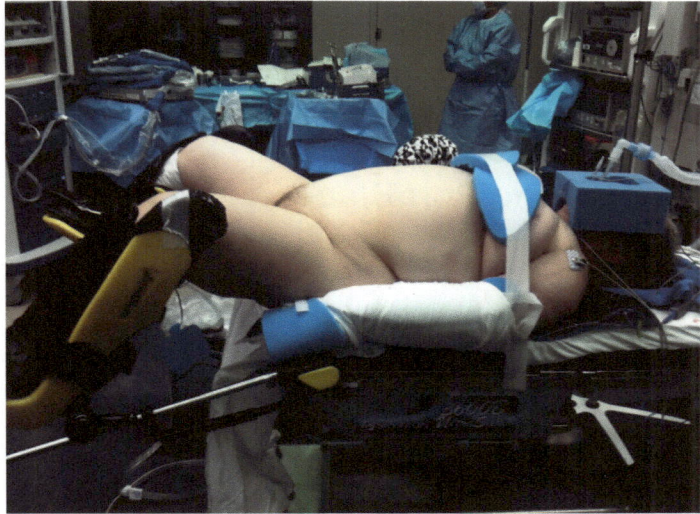

Figure 2: Patient positioning in modified dorsal lithotomy position.

This author prefers the RUMI™ system (Fig. **3**). Figure of eight sutures of an absorbable material such as polyglactin 910 (Ethicon Endosurgical, Somerville, NJ, USA) is placed at 3 o'clock and 9 o'clock on the cervix. This allows the operator or his/her assistant to use the sutures as traction to remove the uterus vaginally aided by an inflated balloon inside the uterus.

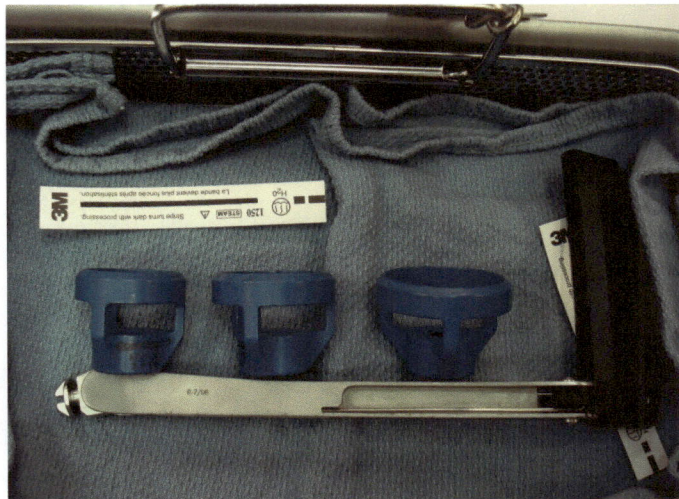

Figure 3: The RUMI system of uterine manipulation with reusable colpotomy rings and manipulator.

Trocar Placement

Pneumoperitoneum is established by either inserting a Veress needle into the abdomen or via direct trocar insertion under laparoscopic guidance. In a patient with a prior laparotomy, a preferable point of entry is the left upper quadrant midclavicular point (Palmer's point). Once pneumoperitoneum is established, a reference point of the anterior superior iliac spine is used. Three to five cm in a line directly cephalad from this reference point in the left lower quadrant will be the position of the left hand port or the bipolar device. This puts the trocar site at least 4 cm lateral to the course of the inferior epigastric vessels.

A similar point on the right side will be used for the port for the third instrument arm with a grasper or a retracting device inserted. In the right upper quadrant the port for the second instrument arm is placed. Finally, the camera port is placed either in the supra umbilical fold or up to 4 cm above the umbilicus. There should be at least 10 cm spacing between the distal tip of the endoscope to the target organ and at least 10 cm between the instrument arms or between instrument arms and camera arm (Figs. **4** to **7**). This port placement model prevents external instrument arm collision allowing for full range of motion for all instruments including the camera.

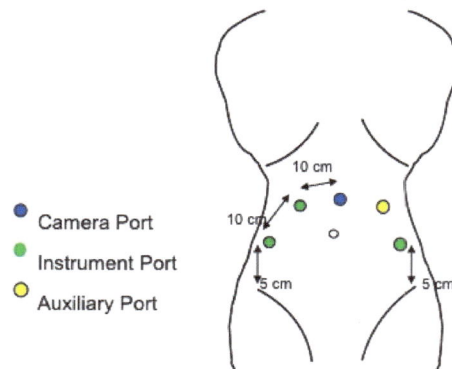

Figure 4: Robotic surgery port placement schematic. Blue = Camera Port Site, green = Robotic Instrument Port Site, Yellow = Auxliary or Assistant Port Site.

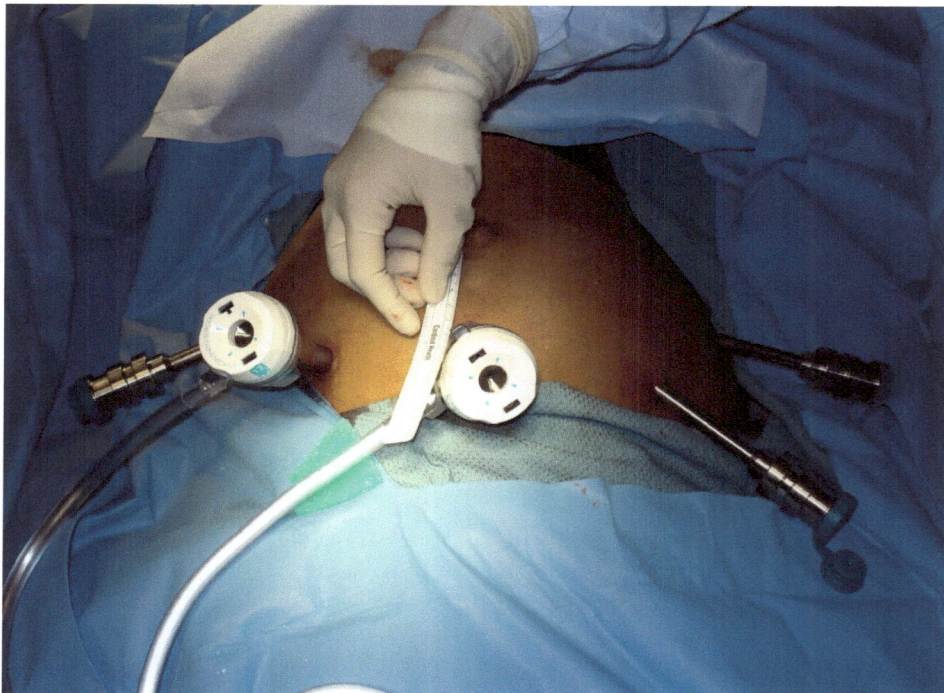

Figure 5: Establishing the port sites after pneumoperitoneum.

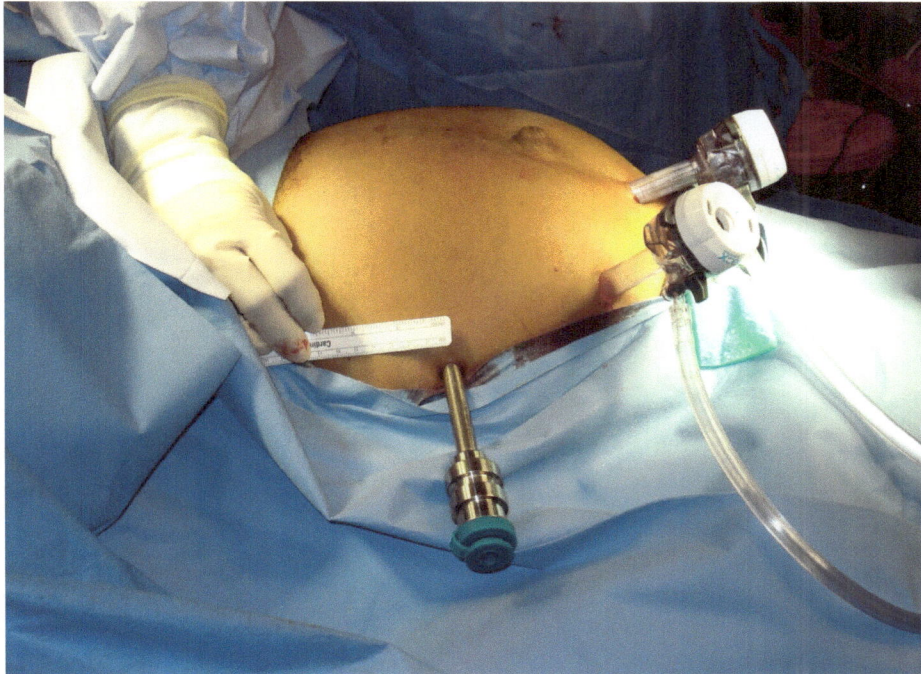

Figure 6: Left lower quadrant robotic instrument port approximately 4 – 5 cm directly cephalad from the anterior superior iliac spine.

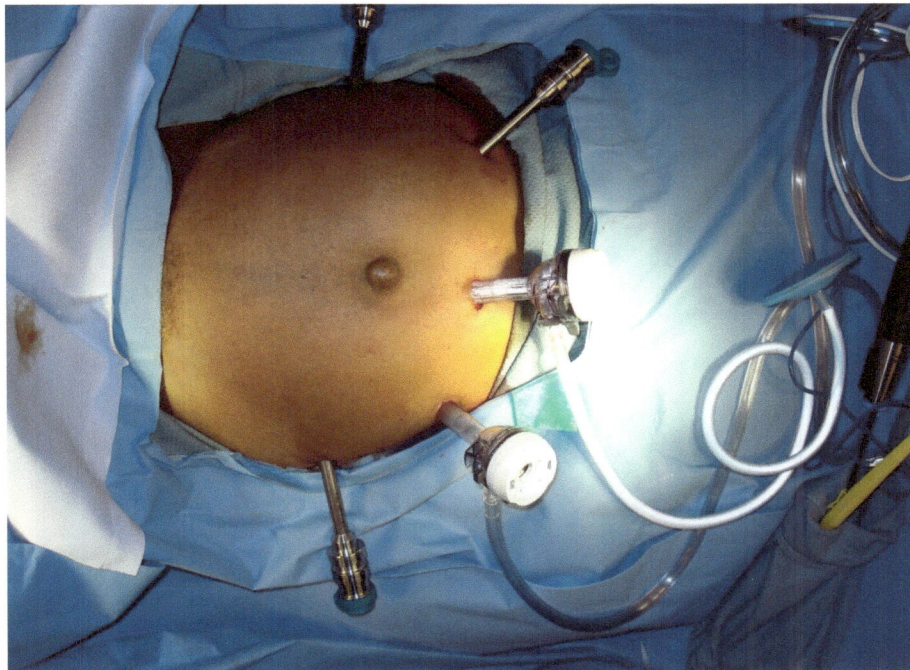

Figure 7: Port Placement.

Prior to placing the left upper quadrant assistant port, the operator should verify that an oral-gastric tube is in situ and under suction to decompress the stomach. Bowel prep may be administered eighteen to twenty four hours prior to the operation in addition to an antiemetic. The use of an antiemetic 24 hours prior to the operation reduces the incidence of postoperative nausea and vomiting in the postoperative period [12]. The pelvis is then visualized and if necessary adhesiolysis performed to restore normal anatomical relationships prior to starting the hysterectomy Video **1**.

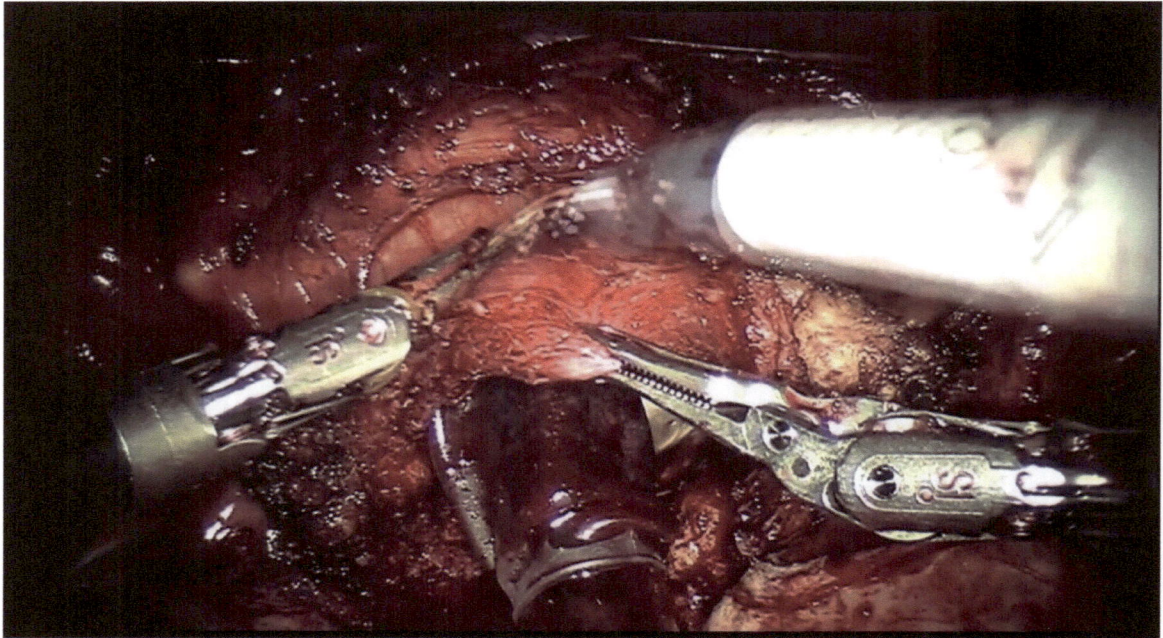

Video 1

Operative Technique

Although most hysterectomies performed either abdominally or laparoscopically begin by transecting the round ligament, it may be helpful to leave the round ligament intact. This helps to provide a reference point if the anatomy is distorted by multiple leiomyomas or pelvic adhesions. It also provides a mechanism for counter-traction when entering the retroperitoneal space. The retroperitoneal space may be entered in an avascular triangle (Video **2**) bounded by the external iliac vessels, the ovarian vessels and the round ligament (Fig. **8**). The ureters are identified in this space. Similarly with the ovarian vessels that can be safely ligated if needed (Fig. **9**). A safe approach to hysterectomy should involve identifying the course of the ureters and skeletonizing the vascular pedicles whenever possible. This allows for an efficient energy transfer and vessel sealing while minimizing ureteral injury.

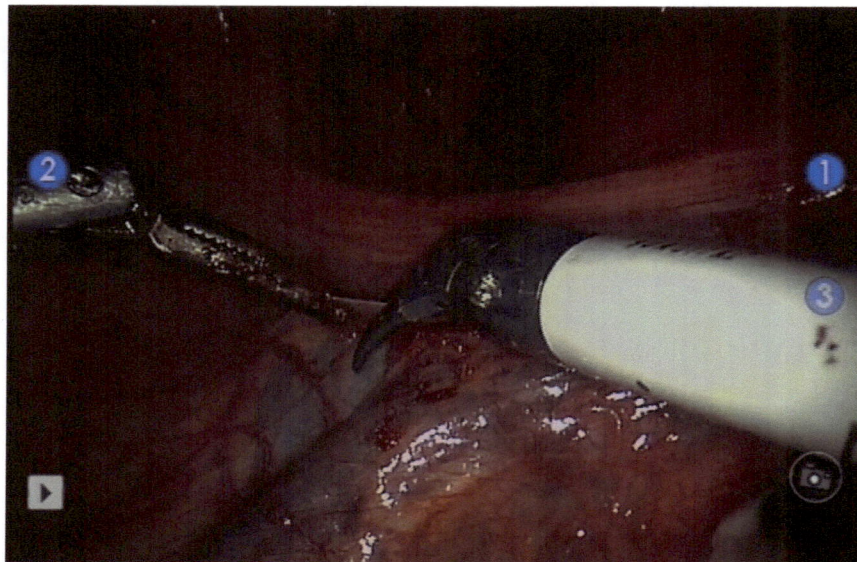

Figure 8: Entering the avascular triangle on the left pelvic sidewall bounded by the round ligament, external iliac vessels and the ovarian vessels.

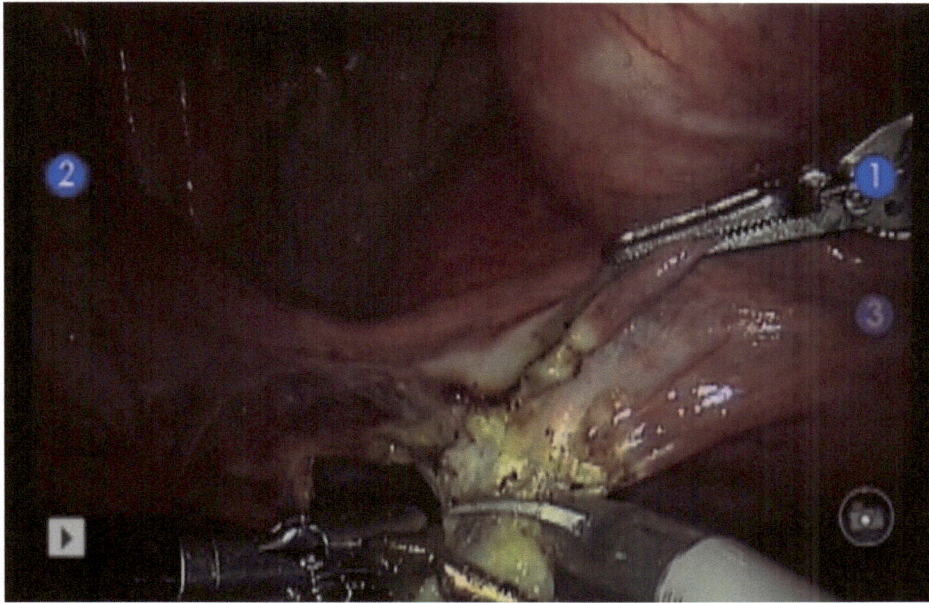

Figure 9: Transecting the proximal aspect of the left utero-ovarian ligament and fallopian tube. Prograsp ™ holding the cut margin of the fallopian tube and providing retraction medially.

After division of the ovarian vessels or the infundibulopelvic ligament, the dissection is continued in a diagonal and medial fashion along the posterior leaf of the broad ligament to the level of the internal os of the cervix (Fig. **10**). This allows exposure of the posterior aspect of the uterine vessels. Now the round ligament can be divided and the dissection on the anterior peritoneal reflection or vesico-uterine fold of visceral peritoneum can be started. It may be necessary to completely expose the anterior aspect of the uterine vessels during this part of the dissection instead of trying to fully develop the bladder flap. This is especially important if there are large anterior lower segment myomas that obscure the view of the anterior cul-de-sac. The goal of this part of the dissection is to quickly identify and seal all the vascular supply to the uterus with minimal bleeding (Figs. **11** and **12**). This technique allows the operator to minimize conversions when removing large uterus [13].

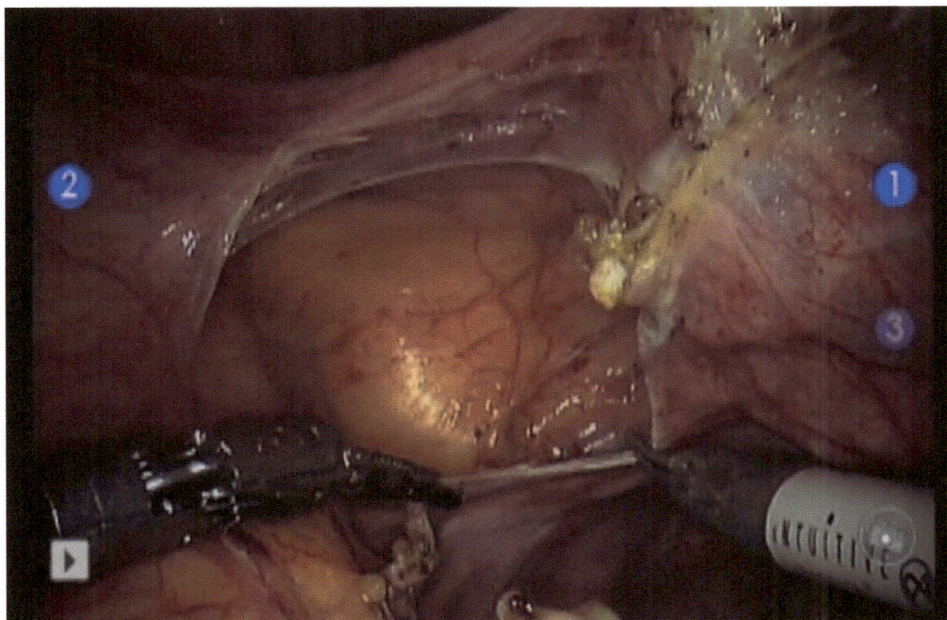

Figure 10: Dividing the posterior leaf of the left broad ligament to expose the uterine vessels posteriorly.

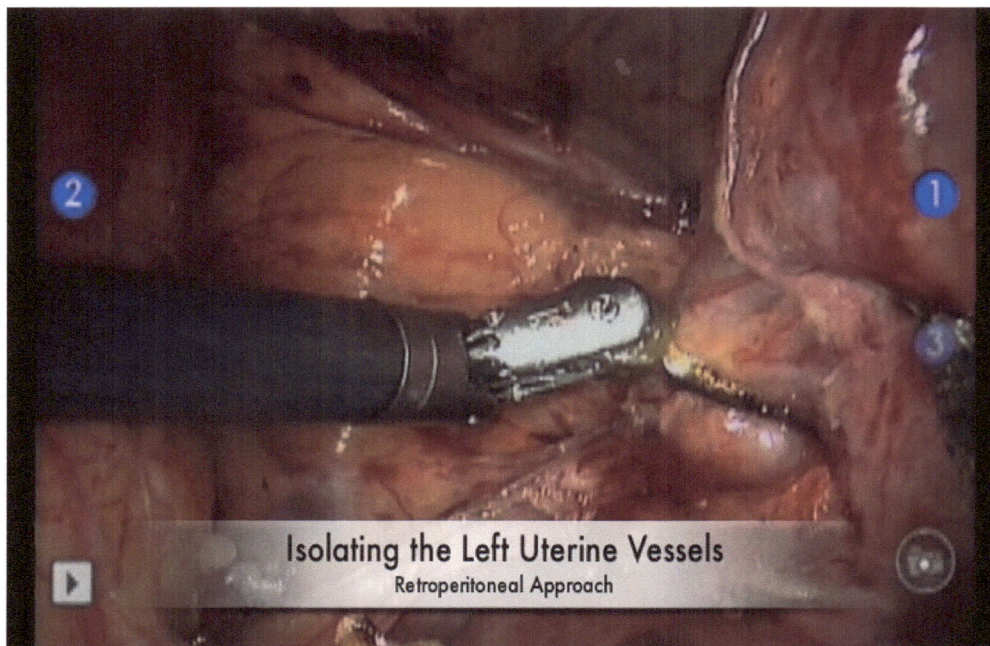

Figure 11: Isolating and sealing the left uterine vessels.

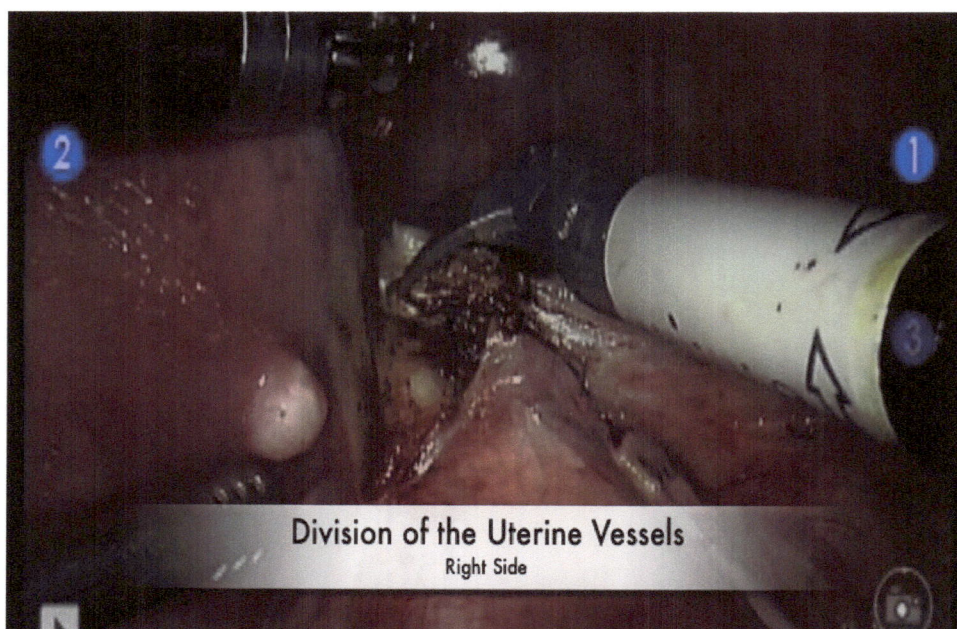

Figure 12: Sealing and dividing the right uterine vessels with the PK Dissector® and Hot Shears ™.

The use of the robotic 4th arm with either an atraumatic grasper or a tenaculum facilitates the manipulation of the specimen in lieu of the external uterine manipulator especially for large uterus. This complements the work of the patient side assistant. When using the 4th arm for retraction, the arm should be wristed away from the operative field of dissection in order to minimize instrument arm collisions internally. After securing the vascular supply to the uterus, the colpotomy incision is made. It is often better to start the incision on the posterior aspect of the colpotomy ring since the rectum and both uterosacral ligaments can be readily identified without any additional dissection (Figs. **13** and **14**). This may not be feasible when the posterior cul-de-sac is obliterated as in the case of Stage IV endometriosis.

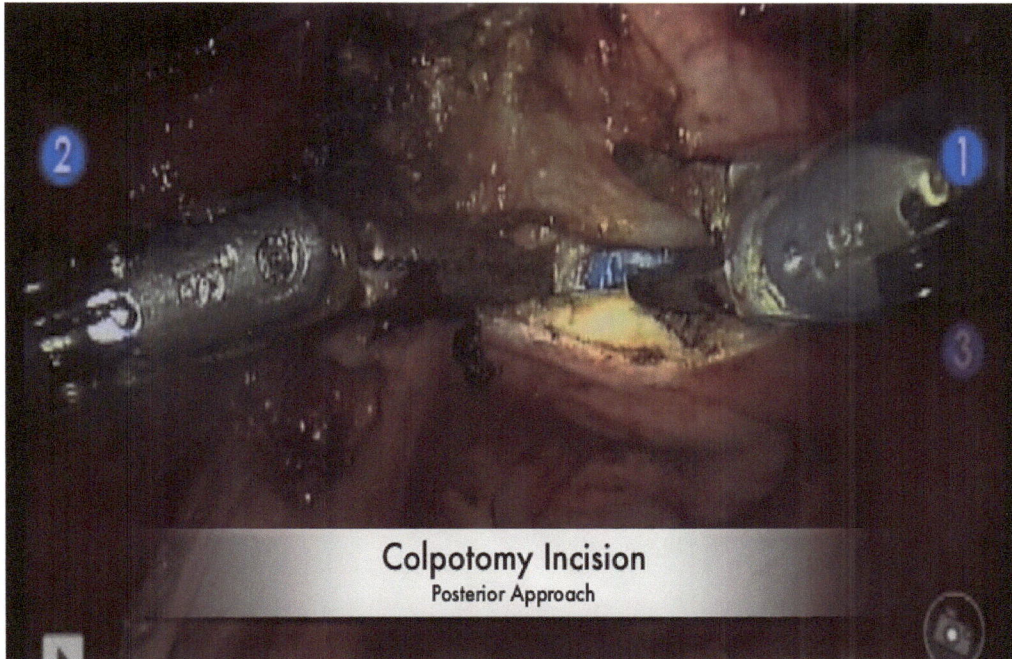

Figure 13: Colpotomy incision in between the uterosacral ligaments.

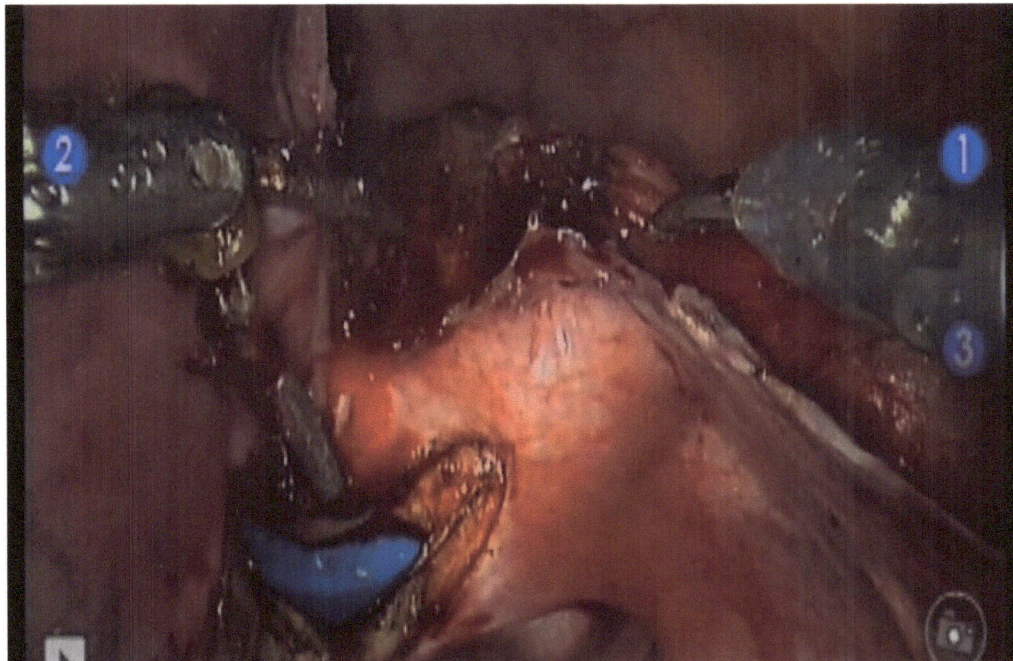

Figure 14: Colpotomy incision maintaining the insertion of the cardinal-uterosacral ligaments – right side.

Performing the colpotomy incision anteriorly requires complete mobilization of the bladder flap leaving at least one to two cm of healthy vagina for the closure of the vaginal cuff. The default energy settings on the PK Dissector may be used and the setting on the HotShears™ should not exceed 35 watts to minimize excessive thermal injury to the vagina. The edges of the vagina may become devitalized or necrotic by using excessive thermal energy and this has been attributed as a cause for post-hysterectomy vaginal cuff dehiscence [14]. When making the colpotomy incision, the tissue should be placed on tension for optimal results.

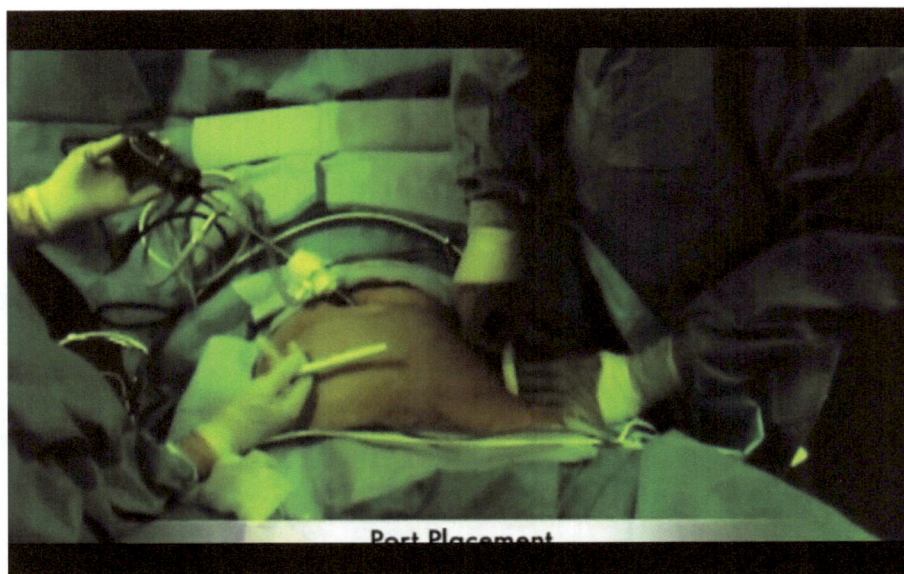

Video 2

Specimen Removal

The specimen can be removed in a number of ways. It can be delivered through the vagina and if necessary morcellated trans-vaginally. It can also be removed using a mechanical device inserted through one of the abdominal trocar sites. Closure of the vaginal cuff is accomplished using the same techniques as open abdominal hysterectomy. In fact, the entire robotic hysterectomy can be considered an open surgery through a laparoscopic access.

Vaginal closure should include the insertion of the cardinal-uterosacral ligaments on the vagina. Placing angle sutures as described in the Modified McCall's culdoplasty helps to prevent vault prolapse post-operatively Video **3**. The abdomen can then be thoroughly irrigated. Prior to closing the abdominal skin incisions, a diagnostic cystoscopy can be performed to verify the integrity of the ureters after intravenous injection of Indigo Carmine dye.

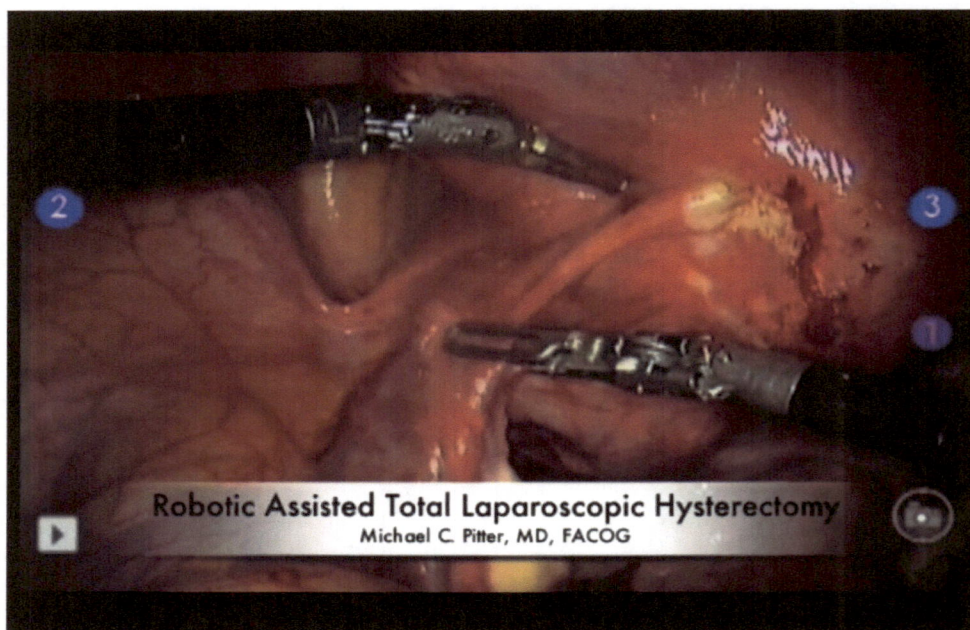

Video 3

OUTCOMES

Robotic Assisted Laparoscopic Hysterectomy may be indicated for complicated procedures that would be normally performed by open abdominal approach. A recent study showed that robotically assisted surgery allowed its use in patients with complex pathology in whom conventional laparoscopy could be difficult and limited [13]. Operative times and estimated blood loss appear to decrease with increasing experience with robotic surgery perhaps at a different rate from that seen with traditional laparoscopy [15 – 17]. In addition, women with large uteri may successfully undergo robotically assisted hysterectomy with low morbidity, low blood loss and minimal risk of conversion to laparotomy [13] Table **2**.

Table 2: A chronological review of the major articles published on Robotic Hysterectomy.

Author	No. of Patients	Mean Age (yrs)	Operative Time (mins)	EBL (ml)	Weight of Specimen (gms)	BMI	LOS (days)	Conversions (%)	Complications	(%) Rate of Complications	AAGL Classification
Diaz-Arrastia et al.	11	55	420	300	Not Reported	29.8	2	0	Bleeding from IP	9.1	II B
Reynolds et al.	16	41	242	73	131.5	27.8	1.5	0	Vaginal Cuff Hematoma, Thermal Injury to the bowel, pneumonia	18.7	III (4), IVE (12)
Advincula et al.	6	40	254	87.5	121.7	26	1.3	0	Vaginal Cuff Hematoma	16.7	IVE (3) III (1)
Fiorentino et al.	20	43	192	81	98	23.1	2	10	Vaginal Cuff Hematoma	5	IVE (18)
Kho et al.	91	50	128	79	135.5	50.3	1.3	0	Ileus, cuff abscess, pneumonia, exacerbation of CHF	7.7	IVE (91)
Payne et al.	100	43	119	61	216	28.8	1.1	4	Cystotomy, Vaginal Cuff Infection	2	IVE (100)
Boggess et al.	152	47	122.9	79	347	30.7	1.1	0	Vaginal Cuff Hematoma, UTI, Left Ureteral Injury, Cuff Abscess, Small Bowel Enterotomy	5.6	IVE (152)
Payne, Pitter et al.	256	46	151.4	98.9	574.5	31.1	1.1	1.6	Pulmonary Embolism, Vaginal Cuff Dehiscence, Injury to the Bladder	3.5	III, IVE

One major limitation with this technology is the lack of haptics or tactile feedback. This can be overcome by training and experience and be replaced with "visual haptics"; a concept of using visual cues to determine relative tissue deflection in response to pressure. Other concerns regarding the cost of the equipment are still to be reconciled especially in today's economy. We are awaiting additional well designed studies to more closely examine the technique of robotic hysterectomy. In any event, current information suggests that it is a safe and reproducible method of addressing benign gynecologic pathology.

REFERENCES

[1]   Jacoby VL, Autry A, Jacobson G, Domush R, Nakagawa S, Jacoby A. Nationwide Use of Laparoscopic Hysterectomy Compared With Abdominal and Vaginal Approaches. Obst Gynecol 2009; 114: 1041-8.

[2]   Thomson Reuters Solucient Data 2008 – 2009.

[3]   Reich H, Decaprio J, McGlynn F. Laparoscopic hysterectomy. J Gynecol Surg 1989; 5: 213–216.

[4]   Farquhar CM, Steiner CA. Hysterectomy rates in the United States 1990-1997. Obstet Gynecol 2002; 99: 229-34.

[5]   Schurr MO, Buess G, Nelsius B, Voges U. Robotics and telemanipulation technologies for endoscopic surgery. A review of the ARTEMIS project. Advanced Robotic Telemanipulator for Minimally Invasive Surgery. Surg Endosc 2000 May; 14(5): 417-8.

[6]   Reynolds RK, Advincula AP. Robot-assisted laparoscopic hysterectomy: technique and initial experience. Am J Surg 2006; **191**: 555–560.

[7]   Wu JM, Wechter ME, Geller EJ, Nguyen TV, Visco AG. Hysterectomy rates in the United States, 2003. Obstet Gynecol 2007;110: 1091–5.

[8]   Olive DL, Parker WH, Cooper JM, Levine RL. The AAGL classification system for laparoscopic hysterectomy. Classification committee of the American Association of Gynecologic Laparoscopists. J Am Assoc Gynecol Laparosc 2000; 7: 9–15.

[9]   Cadiere GB, Himpens J, Germay O, *et al.* Feasibility of robotic laparoscopic surgery: 146 cases. World J Surg 2001; 25: 1467–77.

[10]   Diaz-Arrastia C, Jurnalov C, Gomez G, Townsend C Jr. Laparoscopic hysterectomy using a computer-enhanced surgical robot. Surg Endosc 2002; 16: 1271–3.

[11]   Advincula AP, Reynolds RK. The use of robot-assisted laparoscopic hysterectomy in the patient with a scarred or obliterated anterior cul-de-sac. JSLS 2005; **9**: 287–291.

[12]   Gan TJ, Franiak R, Reeves J. Ondansetron Orally Disintegrating Tablets Versus Placebo for the Prevention of Postdischarge Nausea and Vomiting After Ambulatory Surgery. Anesth Analg 2002; 94:1199-1200.

[13]   Payne TP, Dauterive FR, Pitter MC, Giep HN, Giep BN, Grogg TW, Shanbour A, Goff D, Hubert H. Robotically Assisted Hysterectomy in Patients With Large Uteri: Outcomes in Five Community Practices. Obstet Gyncol 2010;115:535-42.

[14]   Kho, Rosanne M.; Akl, Mohamed N.; Cornella, Jeffrey L.; Magtibay, Paul M.; Wechter, Mary Ellen; Magrina, Javier F. Incidence and Characteristics of Patients With Vaginal Cuff Dehiscence After Robotic Procedures. Obstet Gynecol. 114(2, Part 1): 231-235, August 2009.

[15]   Pitter MC, Anderson P, Blissett A, Pemberton N. Robotic assisted gynaecological surgery-establishing training criteria; minimizing operative time and blood loss. Int J Med Robot 2008; 4: 114–20.

[16]   Lenihan JP Jr, Kovanda C, Seshadri-Kreaden U. What is the learning curve for robotic assisted gynecologic surgery? J Minim Invasive Gynecol 2008; 15: 589–94.

[17]   Payne TN, Dauterive FR. A comparison of total laparoscopic hysterectomy to robotically assisted hysterectomy: surgical outcomes in a community practice. J Minim Invasive Gynecol 2008; 15: 286–91.

CHAPTER 5

Robot-Assisted Tubal Anastomosis: The Evolution, Technique and Outcomes

Sejal Patel* and Nora Algothani

Center for Reproductive Medicine, 3435 Pinehurst Ave, Orlando, FL 32803

Abstract: Robotic assisted surgery is an emerging technology that has expanded the armamentarium of minimally invasive surgeons including the reproductive surgeons. Tubal anastomosis is among the procedures that have been done with robotic assistance. Robotic technology bridges the benefits of open microsurgery through a laparoscopic approach. This review will describe the evolution of robotic technology, the instrumentation and the essential components in the system. The technique of a robotic assisted tubal anastomosis is discussed.

INTRODUCTION

Worldwide, more than 153 million women have chosen sterilization as their contraceptive method [1]. As many as 20% will subsequently express regret due to a change in family circumstances such as the death of a child, improved economic situation or change in marital status [2]; 1-5% of these patients will request sterilization reversal [1,3,4]. For couples that desire fertility after tubal ligation, only two options are available including surgical tubal anastomosis or *in vitro* fertilization. For those who choose surgical sterilization reversal, the procedure can be performed through a laparotomy, laparoscopy or robotic approach.

History

Laparoscopic surgery was first implemented by gynecologists the 1970's [5]. Compared to laparotomy, it has some advantages including decreased adhesion formation [6]. The benefits of laparoscopic surgery are often compromised by a steep learning curve for surgeons, two dimensional vision, limited range of motion [4 degrees of movement], and counterintuitive movements with laparoscopic tools. Surgeons also suffer from ergonomic effects including pain and numbness in the upper extremities during lengthy procedures [7, 8].

The introduction of robotic technology encompasses all the benefits of minimally invasive surgery while solving many of those limitations. Robotics offers three dimensional vision, improved ergonomics, tremor reduction, and intra-abdominal dexterity with seven degrees of articulation.

ROBOTIC SYSTEMS UTILIZED IN GYNECOLOGY

To date three functional robotics systems have been utilized in gynecological surgery. The first surgical robot was the automated endoscope system for optimal positioning [AESOP]. This robotic system is designed to hold and control the laparoscopic camera.

The Zeus surgical system is one of two telerobotic systems developed by Computer Motion in the early 1990. It was subsequently purchased by Intuitive Surgical, the producer of the da Vinci surgical system. The Zeus system contains two separate subsystems, the "surgeon-side" and the "patient-side". It was then modified to include three-dimensional vision and improved intra-abdominal dexterity [e.g. MicroWrist] [9].

The da Vinci robotic system received FDA approval in 2000 for use intra-abdominal surgeries. It consists of three components; a patient side surgical cart, a stereoscopic vision system, and the surgeon console. The surgical cart contains four robotic arms that connect to the laparoscopic trocars. The surgeon operates the robotic arms by maneuvering master controls at the console [10]. Each laparoscopic instrument has seven degree of freedom for intra-abdominal articulation. The console contains binoculars through which the surgeon views the operation in three-dimensional vision [10].

*Address correspondence to Sejal Dharia Patel: Center for Reproductive Medicine, 3435 Pinehurst Ave, Orlando, FL 32803; email: reipatel@aol.com

Togas Tulandi and Arnold Advincula (Eds)

Preliminary studies at the University of Michigan demonstrating the efficacy and safety of the da Vinci in robotic assisted hysterectomies and myomectomies led to FDA approval for its use in gynecology in 2005 [11]. This system is now the only commercially available robotic system approved for gynecological surgery. In addition to the original prototype, two other da Vinci surgical systems are now commercially available. The da Vinci S-series, is a slimmer model decreasing the bulkiness of the robot. The da Vinci S HD incorporates an integrated touch screen monitor, telestration for enhanced teaching and team communication, as well as a TilePro multi-input display that incorporates an integrated view of patient critical information (e.g. radiographic images superimposed on the operative field).

TUBAL ANASTOMOSIS

Laparotomy

In 1977, Gomel [12] first utilized microsurgical technique for tubal anastomosis and reported improved outcomes as compared to macro surgery. The reported pregnancy rates [PR] were 30-63% at 6 months and 53-80% at 12 months [13].

Laparoscopy

The first laparoscopic unilateral sterilization reversal using biologic glue with intraluminal guidance was first reported by Sedbon *et al.* in 1989. The pregnancy rates were poor [14]. In 1992, Koh and Janik applied the principles of microsurgery for laparoscopic tubal anastomosis [13]. The pregnancy rates improved overtime [15-19]. In a large retrospective study, Yoon *et al.* [17] reported that among 202 cases of laparoscopic tubal anastomosis, the pregnancy rates were 60 %, 79.4%, and 83.3 % at 6, 12, and 18 months respectively. The results are comparable to those by open microsurgery [19]. The study also reported that after 15 cases, the operative times for bilateral anastomosis decreased from 4 hours to an average of 2 hours.

Many authors re-approximate the muscularis layer with four interrupted sutures at the 3, 6, 9, and 12 positions and close the serosa with 2-3 interrupted sutures [13, 17]. Others used one stitch technique [15], two stitch technique [16], or three stitch technique [20] closing both muscularis and serosal layers. Laparoscopic tubal anastomosis offers the benefits of minimally invasive surgery. However, it is limited by the absence of stereoscopic vision, difficulty with intra-abdominal suturing and handling fine suture with laparoscopic instruments [13, 15, 19].

Robotic

The feasibility of robotic assisted tubal anastomosis was first tested in 1998 in animal models using the Zeus system [21]. This was followed by a pilot study in women [22]. The procedure was successfully completed in all patients without complications. The mean operative time to complete bilateral anastomosis was 159+/- 33.8 minutes. The pregnancy rates at 6 and 12 month follow up were 89% and 50% respectively. Subsequently, Goldberg *et al.* compared tubal anastomosis using the same system with conventional laparoscopic approach and found similar results [23]. The procedure was performed by placing four 8-0 polyglactin sutures at 3, 6, 9, and 12 o'clock. The operative time of robotic procedure, however was longer [>2 hr].

Using the da Vinci robotic system, Degueldre *et al.* [24] reported comparable operating times to that of open microsurgery. Two of their 8 patients conceived at 4 months following the surgery. Other reports then followed [25-28]. The largest series consisted of 97 cases of robotic assisted tubal anastomosis [28]. The overall pregnancy and live birth rates were 71% and 62% respectively.

ROBOTIC TUBAL ANASTOMOSIS

The Candidate

The ideal candidates for tubal reversal are those who have normal ovulatory function, seminal parameters and intrauterine anatomy. Gordts *et al.* performed microsurgical tubal anastomosis by minilaparotomy and found that the pregnancy rates among those who had had sterilization using a clip or ring were 72-78% [29]. The results of robotic tubal anastomosis are expected to be similar.

The Procedure

The set up includes the use of a surgical table with a gel pad placed under the patient and used to stabilize an inflatable bean bag. The patient's shoulders and abdomen are positioned in the middle of the bean bag, and the patient is placed in a low lithotomy position with the knees in the same plane as the pelvic girdle. The elbows, shoulders and chest are cushioned and then the position is taped to the table to prevent movement in steep trendelenberg (Fig. **1**). Consistent intrauterine manipulation is important to allow for chromopertubation during the anastomosis. We use a V care uterine manipulation system. Any reliable uterine manipulator with the capability to chromotubate is sufficient.

Patient Positioning

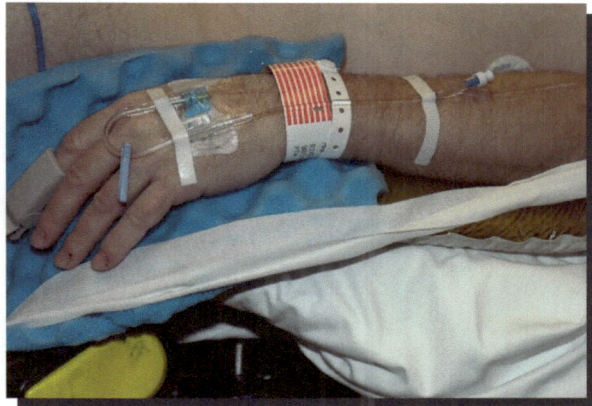

- B: Arms padded with gel and foam and then the position is taped.

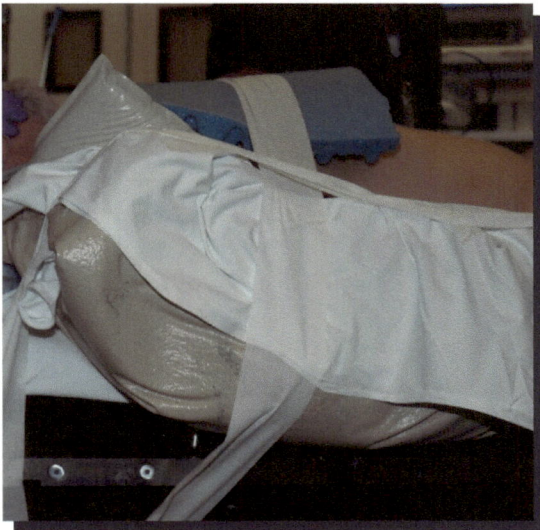

- A: Patient is positioned supine on the beanbag which when inflated around shoulder will act as a harness

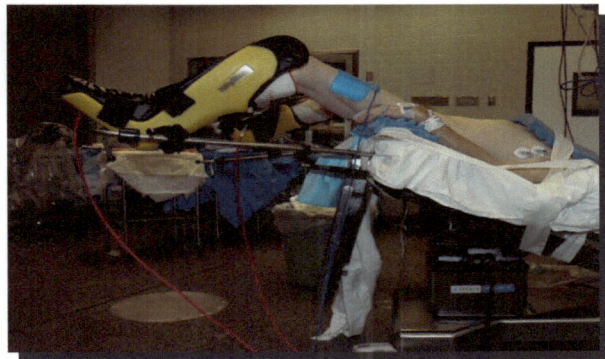

- C: Steep trendelenberg position which is at a 45° angle with bed at lowest point the floor

Figure 1: The patient is positioned on a inflatable bean bag which is positioned on a jelly like pad to prevent movement in steep trendelenberg. The bean bag is inflated around the shoulders and sides to support the patient in the appropriate position and then this position is taped to the table to prevent further movement.

Positioning of the Robotic Surgical System

We use a Veress needle for pneumoperitoneum before inserting a 12 mm primary trocar at the level of the umbilicus. Two lateral 8 mm da Vinci® ports are placed in the mid-axillary line two centimeters below the level of the umbilicus and separated by a minimum of 8 cm between the port sites (Fig. **2**). After confirming the feasibility of tubal anastomosis, an accessory 8 mm port is placed on the left side between the primary port and the lateral port for irrigation, and for introduction and retrieval of suture material. The robot is then positioned at the left knee (also known as side docking) to provide vaginal access for chromopertubation (Fig. **3**). The robotic arms are then connected to the respective ports.

Robotic Tubal Reversal

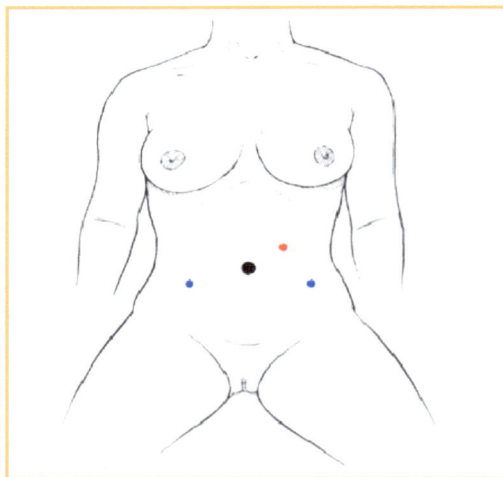

- Umbilicus holds a 12 mm Trocar

- Lateral ports hold a 7 mm da Vinci trocar

- Red accessory port hold a 8mm trocar

Figure 2: Typical port placement for a robotic tubal reversal. The umbilicus houses the robotic camera trocar, with two 8 mm da Vinci trocars approximately 10 cm lateral and 2 cm inferior to the umbilical port. An assistant trocar [8 mm—disposable] is placed for irrigation, suture placement and removal 10 cm lateral and 2 cm superior to the right lateral trocar.

Pregnancy outcomes in the literature

Author/Year	Patients	Patency by HSG (unilateral)	Pregnancy (time)
Degueldre et al, 2009	97	100%	66/97 (47 months)
Patel et al, 2008	18	100%	11/18 (8.9 months)
Falcone et al, 2007	26	NA	16/26 (9 months)
Vlahos et al 2007	5	Ns	2/5
Falcone et al, 2000	10	100%	5/10 (12 months)

Degueldre et al, 2009

Figure 3: The Da Vinci surgical tower is positioned in the center of the left knee at an angle to allow for intraoperative vaginal access for chromopertubation purposes.

Technique of Anastomosis

Instruments for robotic assisted tubal anastomosis include a Black Diamond Microforceps and Potts scissors to strip the serosa off the distal segment (Video **1**). The tip is then resected exposing the distal lumen (Video **2**). Using a Micro Bipolar instrument the mesosalpinx of the proximal segment is cauterized and transected (Video **3**). The proximal segment is mobilized and the tip transected demonstrating the proximal lumen (Video **4**). Chromopertubation is utilized to demonstrate patency of the proximal tubal segment (Video **5**). The mesosalpinx is then reapproximated with 1-2 interrupted 6-0 polyglactin sutures. The mucosal and muscular layers of the tubal segments are sutured with two to four interrupted 7-0 polyglactin sutures (Videos **6** and **7**). The serosa was closed separately with a running 7-0-polygalactin suture and patency of the surgical repair was determined by chromopertubation (Video **8**). Hysteroscopic tubal cannulation Novy cannula can be performed if needed.

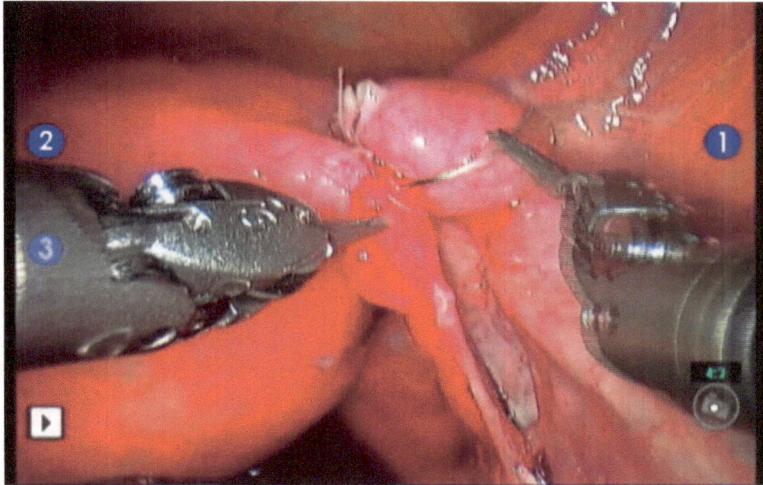

Video 1: Stripping of the distal tubal serosa.

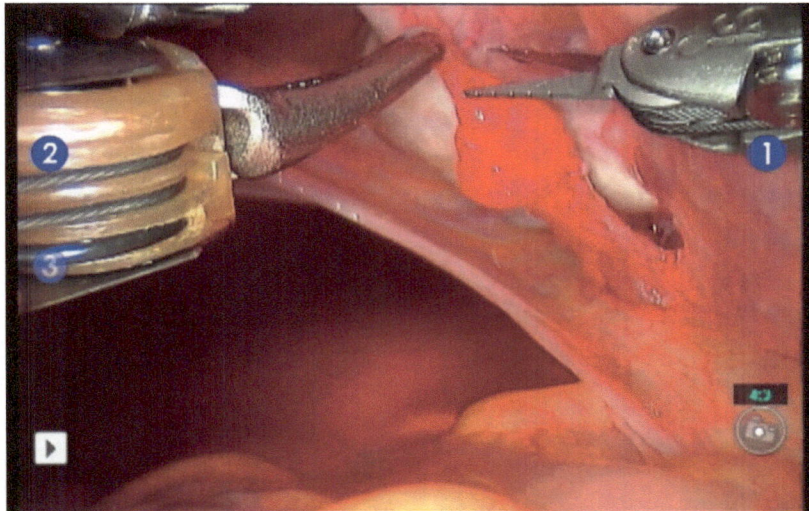

Video 2: Creation of the distal tubal lumen.

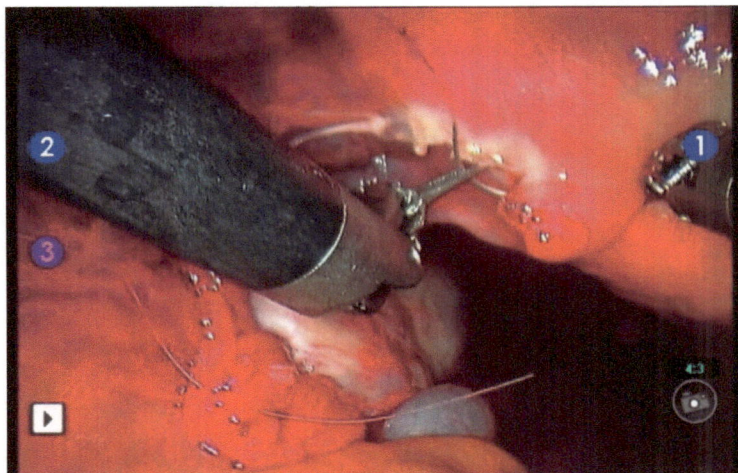

Video 3: Dissection of the mesosalpinx and cautery of the proximal tubal segment.

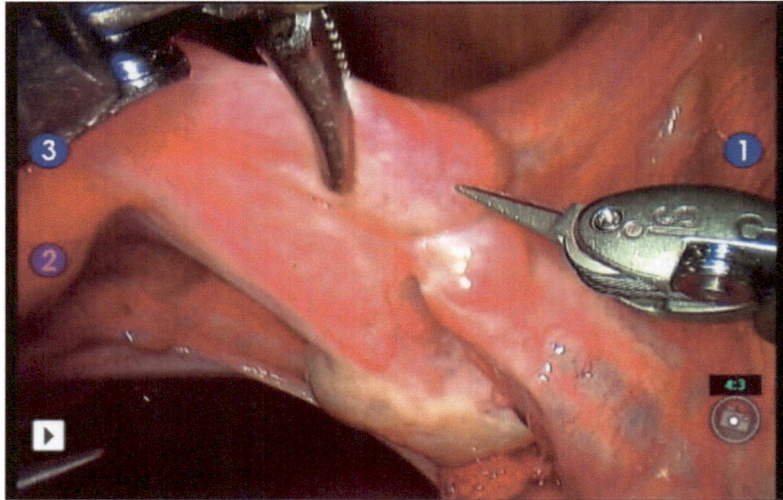

Video 4: Creation of the proximal lumen.

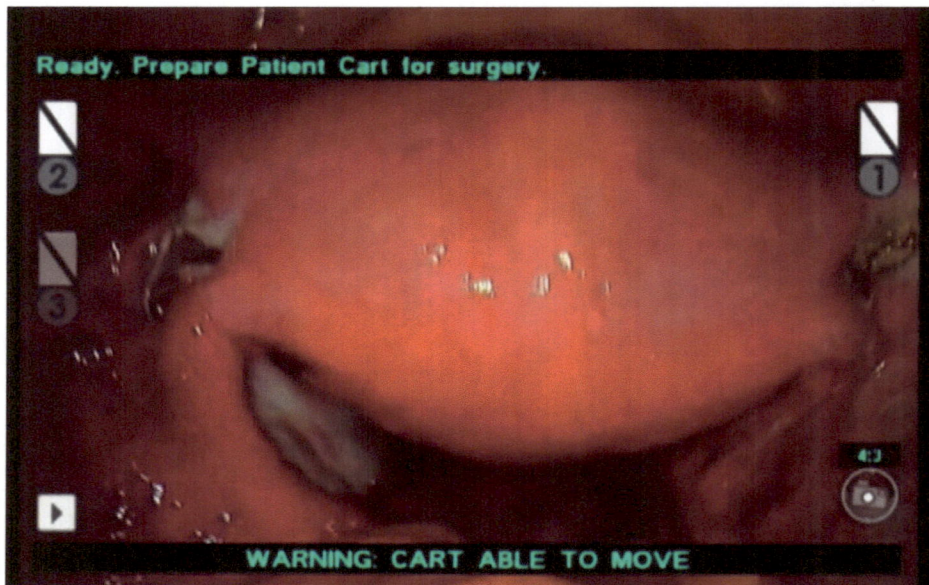

Video 5: Chromopertubation to document proximal tubal patency.

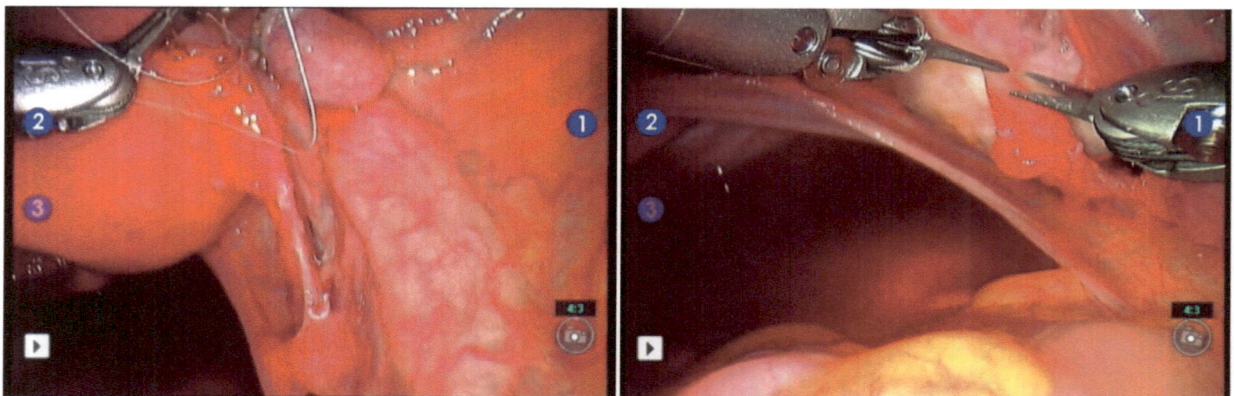

Video 6 & 7: Suturing of the mucosal and muscularis layers of the proximal and distal tubal lumens using 7-0 polyglactin.

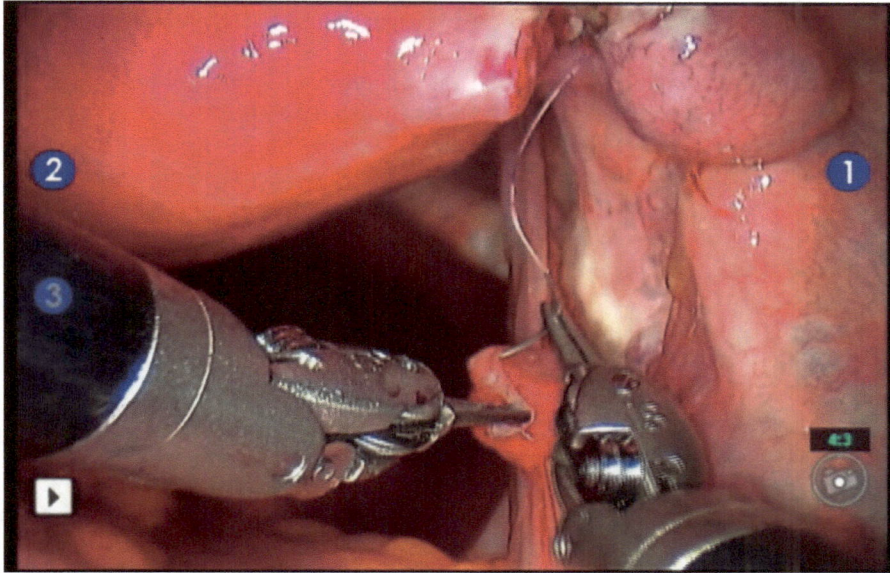

Video 8: Chromopertubation at the completion of the repair to document tubal patency.

Financial Consideration

Two studies demonstrated an increased cost with the robotic procedure as compared to the open approach. Rodgers *et al.* [27] reported a cost difference of $1446 [with the robotic technique being more costly] and Dharia *et al.* $2030.58 [26].

Pregnancy Outcomes

Pregnancy rates after robotic tubal reversal range from 50-71% [23,24,26, 27,29] with ongoing pregnancy rates of 30-62%. Ectopic pregnancy rates range from 11-22% and spontaneous pregnancy loss rates range from 11-26%. The largest series to date consisted of 97 cases of robotic tubal reversal [28]. The average pregnancy rate was 71% with an ongoing pregnancy rate of 62%. Patients aged <35 years had a pregnancy rate of 91%, between the ages of 36-39 years 75%, between the ages of 40-42 years 50%, and those aged >43 had a pregnancy rate of 33%. Most pregnancies occurred in the first 6 months after surgery [28].

ROLE OF TUBAL ANASTOMOSIS IN THE ERA OF IVF

Some authors advocate that *in vitro* fertilization [IVF] should be the first line of therapy for any patient with tubal damage [30]. The American Society of Reproductive Medicine IVF-monitoring study reports pregnancy rates at 36.5% per IVF cycle, with higher pregnancy rates up to 60% in certain centers [31, 32]. As previously reviewed, pregnancy rates with sterilization reversal are comparable to those achieved with IVF technology. However, conception due to IVF treatment occurs earlier. Tubal reversal can result in several pregnancies overtime. Yet, it is associated with an increased risk of ectopic gestation and a chance for reocclusion. IVF allows for correction of multiple infertility factors, but it carries the risk of multiple gestation and medication side effects [33]. IVF and tubal reversal could be considered as complementary procedures, and the choice depends on the individual patient [34].

REFERENCES

[1]   UNDP/UNFPA/WHO/World Bank Special Programme of Research, Development and Research Training in Human Reproduction [HRP]. Advances in Female Sterilization Research. World Health Organization--Progress in Reproductive Health Research Newsletter 1995; 36 at http://www.who.int/reproductive-health/hrp/progress/36/news36_1.en.html accessed on 4/13/2009.

[2]   Hillis SD, Marchbanks PA, Tylor LR, Peterson HB. Poststerilization regret: findings from the United States Collaborative Review of Sterilization. Obstet Gynecol 1999; 93: 889-895.

[3]   Spivak MM, Librach CL, Rosenthal DM. Reversal of sterilization: a six year study. Am J Obstet Gynecol 1986; 154: 355-361.

[4]   Divers WA Jr. Characteristics of women requesting reversal of sterilization. Fertil Steril 1984; 41: 233-236

[5]   Siegler, AV; Berenyi, KJ. Laparoscopy in gynecology. Obstet Gynecol 1969; 34:572-5.

[6]   Adamyan, LV. Minimally invasive surgery in gynecologic practice. Int J Gynecol Obstet 2003; 82: 347-355.

[7]   Berguer R, Forkey DL, Smith WD. Ergonomic problems associated with laparoscopic surgery. Surg Endosc 1999; 13: 466-468.

[8]   Kano N, Yamakawa T, Kasugai H. Laparoscopic surgeon's thumb. Arch Surg 1993; 128:1172.

[9]   Marescaux J, Rubino F. The Zeus robotic system: experimental and clinical applications. Surg Clin N Am 2003; 83: 1305-1315.

[10]   Ballantyne GH, Moll F. The da Vinci telerobotic surgical system: the virtual operative field and telepresence surgery. Surg Clin N AM 2003; 83: 1293-1304.

[11]   Advincula AP, Song A, Burke W, Reynolds RK. Preliminary experience with robot-assisted laparoscopic myomectomy. J Am Assoc Gynecol Laparosc 2004; 11: 511-518.

[12]   Gomel, V. Tubal reanastomosis by microsurgery. Fertil Steril 1977; 28:59-65.

[13]   Koh, CH; Janik, GM. Laparoscopic microsurgical tubal anastomosis. Obstet Gynecol Clin N Am 1999; 26: 189-200.

[14]   Sedbon E, Delajoulinieres JB, Boudouris O, et el. Tubal desterilization through exclusive laparoscopy. Hum Reprod 1989; 4: 158-159.

[15]   Dubuisson JB and Swolin K. Laparoscopic tubal anastomosis [the one stitch technique]: preliminary results. Hum Reprod 1995; 10: 2044-2046.

[16]   Reich H, McGlynn F, Parente C, et al. Laparoscopic tubal anastomosis. J Am Assoc Gynecol Laparosc 1993; 1: 16-19.

[17]   Yoon TK, Sung HR, Kang HG, et al. Laparoscopic tubal anastomosis: fertility outcome in 202 cases. Fertil Steril 1999; 72: 1121-1126.

[18]   Dubuisson JB, Chapron C, Nos C, et al. Sterilization reversal : fertility results. Hum Reprod 1995; 10: 1145-1151.

[19]   Barjot PJ, Marie G, Theobold PV. Laparoscopic tubal anastomosis and reversal of sterilization. Hum Reprod 1999; 14: 1222-1225.

[20]   Katz E, Donesky BW. Laparoscopic tubal anastomosis. A pilot study. J Reprod Med 1994; 39: 497-498.

[21]   Margossian H, Garcia-Ruiz A, Falcone T, Goldberg JM, Attaran M, Gagner M. Robotically assisted laparoscopic microsurgical uterine horn anastomosis. Fertil Steril 1998; 70: 530-534.

[22]   Falcone T, Goldberg J, Margossian H, Stevens L. Robotic-assisted laparoscopic microsurgical tubal anastomosis: a human pilot study. Fertil Steril 2000; 73: 1040-1042.

[23]   Goldberg JM, Falcone T. Laparoscopic microsurgical tubal anastomosis with and without robotic assistance. Hum Reprod 2003; 18: 145-147.

[24]   Degueldre M, Vandromme J, Huong PT, Cadiere GB. Robotically assisted laparoscopic microsurgical tubal reanastomosis: a feasibility study. Fertil Steril 2000; 74: 1020-1023.

[25]   Dharia SP, Steinkampf M, Whitten SJ, Malizia BA. Robotically assisted tubal reanastomosis in a Fellowship Training program [abstract]. ESHRE Annual Meeting; Berlin, Germany June 2004.

[26]   Patel SD, Steinkampf M, Whitten SJ, Malizia BA. Robotically assisted tubal sterilization reversal: surgical technique and cost-effectiveness versus conventional surgery [abstract]. American Society for Reproductive Medicine Annual Meeting; Philadelphia, PA, October 2004.

[27]   Rodger AK, Goldberg JM, Hammel JP, et al. Tubal anastomosis by robotic compared with outpatient minilaparotomy. Obstet Gynecol 2007;109:1375–1380

[28]   Caillet M, Vandromme J, Rozenberg S, Paesmans M, Germay O, Degueldre M. Robotically assisted laparoscopic microsurgical tubal reanastomosis: A retrospective study. Fertil Steril 2010; 94(5): 1844-7.

[29]   Gordts S, Campo R, Puttemans P, Gordts S. Clinical factors determining pregnancy outcome after microsurgical tubal anastomosis. Fertil Steril 2009; 92: 1198-1202.

[30]   Holst N, Maltau JM, Forsdahl F, et al. Handling of tubal infertility after introduction of in vitro fertilization: changes and consequences. Fertil Steril 1991; 55: 140-142.

[31]   ASRM/SART Registry (2000) Assisted reproductive technology in the United States: results generated from the American Society for Reproductive Medicine/Society for Assisted Reproductive Technology Registry. Fertil Steril 2000; 72:641-654.

[32]   ASRM/SART Registry (2009) Assisted reproductive technology in the United States: results generated from the American Society for Reproductive Medicine/Society for Assisted Reproductive Technology Registry for the Center for Reproductive Medicine in Orlando, Florida 2009.

[33]   Ribero SC, Tormena RA, Giribela CG, *et al.* Laparoscopic tubal anastomosis. Int J Gynecol Obstet 2004 ; 84 : 142-146.

[34]   Posaci C, Camus M, Osmanagaoglu K, *et al.* Tubal surgery in the era of assisted reproductive technology: clinical options. Hum Reprod 1999; 14: 120-136.

CHAPTER 6

Robotic Surgery in Gynecologic Oncology

Vanna Zanagnolo[1] and Javier F. Magrina[2]*

[1]European Institute of Oncology, Department of Gynaecologic Oncology, Milan, Italy and [2]Mayo Clinic in Arizona, Department of Gynecology, Gynecologic Surgery, Phoenix, AZ

Abstract: The development of robotic technology has facilitated the application of minimally invasive techniques for the treatment and evaluation of patients with gynecologic cancer including early, advanced, and recurrent endometrial, cervical and to a less extent ovarian cancer. Numerous gynecologic oncologists have published their experience using this new technology. Most case series of robotic assisted hysterectomy and lymphadenectomy, as well as radical hysterectomy for cervical cancer show that the procedure is feasible and comparable or superior to laparoscopic surgery. Less common procedures such as robotic radical trachelectomy, radical parametrectomy, and retroperitoneal aortic lymphadenectomy have also been described. Little information is available addressing a robotic approach for the treatment of advanced or recurrent ovarian cancer patients.

Clearly, robotic technology facilitates the surgical approach for endometrial and cervical malignancies as compared to the conventional laparoscopy. Although patient advantages are similar or slightly improved with robotics, there are multiple advantages for the surgeons.

INTRODUCTION

The development of robotic technology has facilitated the application of minimally invasive techniques for the evaluation and treatment of patients with early, advanced, and recurrent endometrial, cervical and ovarian cancer. The use of a robotic system in preset laboratory drills has been associated with faster performance times, increased accuracy, enhanced dexterity, faster suturing, and reduced number of errors when compared to conventional laparoscopic instrumentation [1-4]. Complex operations, such as radical hysterectomy or peri-aortic lymphadenectomy, can be performed in a more efficient fashion. The skills could be acquired in a shorter time but also by a large number of laparotomy surgeons who encountered difficulties with conventional laparoscopy. The application of robotic technology for patients with endometrial, cervical and ovarian cancer will be addressed in this chapter.

ENDOMETRIAL CANCER

We and others have demonstrated a reduction in blood loss, complications, hospital stay, and recovery time without compromising recurrence and survival outcomes in patients with endometrial cancer treated by laparoscopy as compared to laparotomy [5-7]. It is clear that in expert hands laparoscopy should be the standard treatment for these patients. A recent Gynecologic Oncology Group (GOG) prospective randomized trial comparing laparoscopy and laparotomy for endometrial cancer showed that recurrence and survival rates remain unchanged. Accordingly laparoscopy is the standard treatment for endometrial cancer. Despite patient benefits, laparoscopic techniques have remained underutilized, due mainly to a long learning curve and the limitations of the technology as observed in the different settings [8-11].

Robotic technology has reduced the learning curve of minimally invasive procedures and corrected some of the limitations of the laparoscopic technique. This is due to technological advances such as stereoscopic vision, instrument articulation, and laparotomy resemblance of surgical manipulation [2, 3]. The robotic surgical system facilitates suturing and dissection and makes isolation of the vessels, ligation of the uterine arteries, ureteral dissection and lymphadenectomies easier to learn. The techniques resemble more closely conventional open surgery than laparoscopy. As a result, gynecologic oncologists have switched from laparotomy to robotics without laparoscopic training, resulting in a reduction of the number of laparotomy surgeries being performed for gynecologic malignancies [12-14].

---

*Address correspondence to Javier F. Magrina:** Department of Gynecology, Gynecologic Surgery, Mayo Clinic, 5777 East Mayo Boulevard, Phoenix, AZ 85054; Phone: 480-342-2668; Fax: 480-342-2944; E-mail: *jmagrina@mayo.edu*.

In Peiretti's series, the implementation of robotic technology significantly increased the number of endometrial cancer cases treated by a minimally invasive approach in a relatively short period of time [13]. In the 12 months prior to the introduction of robotics surgery, only 22% of endometrial cancer cases were treated by conventional laparoscopy. Whereas in the first 12-month after the implementation of the da Vinci surgical system, 65% of the procedures were robotically assisted, and 35% were laparotomies with no laparoscopies being performed. Their data showed the impact of robotic technology by tripling the number of minimally invasive procedures from the treatment of endometrial cancer during the implementation of the technology.

We performed a prospective analysis of 67 patients undergoing robotic surgery for endometrial cancer between March 2004 and December 2007. Comparison was made with similar patients operated between January 1999 and December 2006 by laparoscopy (37 cases), laparotomy (99 cases) and a combined vaginal/laparoscopic approach (vaginal hysterectomy/laparoscopic lymphadenectomy) (47 cases). The patients were matched by age, body mass index (BMI), histological type and International Federation of Gynecology and Obstetrics (FIGO) staging. The robotic and laparoscopy groups had a similar operating time, reduced blood loss, and shorter hospital stay as compared to laparotomy patients. These results are consistent with other studies of endometrial cancer demonstrating the benefits of minimally invasive surgery (MIS), laparoscopy and robotics, as compared to laparotomy [5-8, 10]. The vaginal group had similar benefits as the laparoscopy and robotic groups but the operating time was longer as compared to laparotomy. This could be due to the double set up and the required time to switch from the vaginal to the laparoscopic portion of the operation.

A summary of perioperative outcomes of robotic surgery for endometrial cancer and comparison between robotic, laparoscopy and laparotomy is demonstrated in Tables **1** to **4** [12-19].

Table 1: Perioperative Outcomes of Robotic Surgery for Endometrial Cancer (Mean Values)

	OR time (min)	EBL (ml)	LN (n)	Hospital Stay (days)	Complications (%)
Gehrig *et al.* [17]					
2008 N=49	189	50	34	1.02	12
Veljovich *et al.* [14]					
2008 N= 25	283	67	18	1.8	8
DeNardis *et al.* [12]					
2008 N=56	177	105	19	1.0	4
Bell *et al.* [15]					
2008 N: 40	184	166	17	2.3	7.5
Boggess *et al.* [16]					
2008 N=103	191	75	33	1.0	6
Seamon *et al.* [19]					
2009 N=105	242	88	31	1.0	13
Peiretti *et al.* [13] 2009 N= 80	173	42	17	2.4	9
Holloway *et al.* [18] 2009 N: 100	171	103	18.7	1.12	3

Table 2: Comparison of Perioperative Outcomes of Robotic, Laparoscopy and Laparotomy Routes for Endometrial Cancer Patients

	TRH	TLH	TAH	P
OR time (min)				
Boggess *et al.* [16]*	191	213	146	<.0001
Mayo AZ**	182	189	163	NS
Bell *et al.* [15]***	184	171	108	.0001

EBL (ml)				
Boggess et al. [16]	75	146	266	<.0001
Bell et al. [15] ***	166	253	317	.01
LN's (n)				
Boggess et al. [16]*	33	23	15	<.0001
Bell et al. [15]***	17	17	15	NS
Hosp. stay (days)				
Boggess et al. [16]*	1.0	1.2	4.4	<.0001
Bell et al. [15]***	2.3	2.0	4.0	.0001
Complications (%)				
Boggess et al. [16]*	6	14	30	(<.0001;.07)**
Bell et al. [15]***	7.5	20	27	(.0015;.03)**

* Robotic=103, Laparoscopy=81, Laparotomy=138; ** Comparing TRH to TAH and TLH respectively; *** Robotic=40, Laparoscopy=30, Laparotomy=40

Table 3: Comparison of Perioperative Outcomes of Robotics and Laparotomy for Endometrial Cancer Patients

	Robotic	Laparotomy	P
OR (min)			
Veljovich et al. [14]*	302	139	<.0001
DeNardis et al. [12]**	177	79	<.0001
EBL (ml)			
Veljovich et al. [14]*	98	197	<.0001
DeNardis et al. [12]**	105	251	<.0001
LNs (n)			
Veljovich et al. [14]*	18	13	NS
DeNardis et al. [12]**	19	18	NS
Hosp Stay (days)			
Veljovich et al. [14]*	1.8	5.3	<.0001
DeNardis et al. [12]**	1.0	3.2	<.0001
Complications (%)			
Veljovich et al. [14]*	8	20.6	NS
DeNardis et al. [12]**	4	20.8	<.001

* Robotic=25,Laparotomy=131; ** Robotic =56, Laparotomy=106

Table 4: Comparison of Perioperative Outcomes of Robotics and Laparoscopy for Endometrial Cancer Patients

	Robotic	Laparoscopy	P
OR min			
Gehrig et al. [17]*	189	215	.0004
Seamon et al. [19]**	242	287	<.001
EBL (ml)			

Gehrig *et al.* [17]*	50	150	<.0001
Seamon *et al.* [19]**	88	200	<.001
LNs (n)			
Gehrig *et al.* [17]*	34	22	.0017
Seamon *et al.* [19]**	31	33	NS
Hosp. Stay (days)			
Gehrig *et al.* [17]*	1.02	1.27	NS
Seamon *et al.* [19]**	1.0	2.0	<.001
Complications (%)			
Gehrig *et al.* [17]*	12	21	NS
Seamon *et al.* [19]**	13	14	NS

* Robotic=49, Laparoscopy=32; ** Robotic=105, Laparoscopy=76

The studies show that robotic technology is preferable to laparoscopy particularly for obese and morbidly obese patients with endometrial cancer. This is related to the shorter operative time, reduced blood loss, increased number of lymph nodes and a shorter hospital stay [15-17]. In our series, we observed a shorter hospital stay for robotic patients as compared to conventional laparoscopy (and also for laparotomy and vaginal/laparoscopy patients), while no differences were observed in terms of operating time, blood loss, or number of lymph nodes. A possible explanation of the discrepancies with other studies could be related to the different laparoscopic experience of the surgeons. Although the initial robotic operating times in some studies (representing the learning curve) are longer as compared to laparotomy, the blood loss is reduced, the hospital stay is shorter, and the number of lymph nodes is similar [12, 14]. In our series the number of pelvic nodes was lower in the robotic group as compared to laparotomy, a difference we did not observe in cervical cancer patients and in ovarian cancer patients [20].

The technological improvements in robotics and as well in laparoscopy have allowed us to obtain similar operating times with these two modalities and also with laparotomy, although this is not shared by others who expressed shorter operating times with laparotomy [12, 14, 16].

We observed similar intra and postoperative complications among the four groups while others have noted reduced postoperative complications in the robotic group as compared to laparotomy [12, 16]. The increased versatility of robotic technology is probably a reason for a significantly lower conversion rate due to complications as compared with laparoscopy.

The use of minimally invasive surgery, robotics or laparoscopy, for patients with endometrial cancer, has been shown to result in a shorter recovery time and improved quality of life without a negative impact on surgical outcome [20, 21]. Despite the evidence favoring minimally invasive surgery for gynecological and non-gynecological cancer patients, there is a lack of general acceptance and application to suitable patients which must be attributed to other factors [5-7, 9, 11, 22]. For laparoscopy, the difficulties with training and instrumentation might be potential factors [4, 22]. For robotics, although with clear surgeon advantages shortening the learning curve, the availability of the robotic system and its cost are major negative factors [23].

CERVICAL CANCER

Early Cervical Cancer

For early cervical cancer, robotic and laparoscopic radical hysterectomy has been shown to have patient advantages over the laparotomy approach. This is due to reduced blood loss, blood transfusions, complications, and length of hospital stay, with the exception of prolonged operating times [9, 24-27]. Similar recurrence and cure rates have been reported when comparing the results of both techniques [9, 24-27]. A prospective randomized trial has under the auspices of the American Association of Gynecologic Laparoscopists comparing minimally invasive radical hysterectomy (laparoscopy or robotics) with laparotomy is presently undergoing [28].

Our surgical approach for the performance of robotic radical hysterectomy has been described elsewhere [29].

Our first robotic radical hysterectomy was performed on April 9 2003. We published our results on 27 patients who underwent robotic radical hysterectomy for the primary treatment of cervical or endometrial cancer at Mayo Clinic Arizona [20]. These patients were compared to two matched groups of patients (laparoscopy, N=31, and laparotomy, N=35) by age, BMI, site and type of malignancy, FIGO staging, uterine size and type of radical hysterectomy. The mean operating time was significantly longer for the laparoscopic (220.4 minutes) group compared to both the robotic (189.9 minutes) and laparotomy (166.8 minutes) groups (p<0.001). The mean blood loss (443 ml; 133 ml; 208 respectively), mean rate of blood loss (2.6 ml; 0.7 ml; 0.9 ml respectively), and mean length of hospital stay (3.6 days; 1.7 days; 2.4 days respectively) were significantly higher for the laparotomy group compared to both the robotic and laparoscopic groups (p<0.05). There were no difference in the number of lymph nodes, and intra or post-operative complications among the three groups. At a mean length of follow up of 31.1 months (range 10-50), none of the patients in the robotic group have experienced recurrence.

Table 5 shows a summary of published perioperative outcomes of robotic surgery for cervical cancer [20, 30-36]. The first published single case report regarding robotic radical hysterectomy was in 2006 [37]. In 2007 a pilot case-control study designed to evaluate the feasibility and efficacy of robotic radical hysterectomy and bilateral pelvic lymph node dissection for early cervical cancer was reported in 7 consecutive patients, compared with 8 patients treated with conventional laparoscopic radical hysterectomy [38]. There were no statistically significant differences observed in the 2 groups regarding operation time (241 vs 300 minutes), number of lymph nodes, and length of resected parametrial tissue, whereas significantly less bleeding (71 vs 160 ml) and shorter hospital stay (4 vs 8 days) were described in the robotic-assisted group (p<0.05).

Table 5: Perioperative Outcomes of Robotic Radical Hysterectomy for Cervical Cancer (Mean Values)

	OR (min)	EBL (ml)	LN (n)	Hospital Stay (days)	Complications (%)
Kim *et al.* [33]					
2008 N= 10	207	355	27.6	7.9	10
Fanning *et al.* [32]					
2008 N=20	6.5 hrs	300	18	1.0	10
Nezhat *et al.* [35]2008 N: 13	323	157	25	2.7	15
Boggess *et al.* [16]					
2008 N=51	210	96	33.8	1.0	7.8
Persson *et al.* [36]					
2009 N= 80	142	150	26	4	10
Maggioni *et al.* [34]					
2009 N=40	272	78	20.4	3.2	5
Magrina *et al.* [20]					
2008 N=27	189	133	25.9	1.7	7
Estape *et al.* [31] 2009 N= 32	2.4 hrs	130	32	2.6	18.8

Laparoscopy and robotics appear preferable to laparotomy for the treatment of early stage cervical cancer. In our hands robotic patients had a shorter operating time, as compared to laparoscopy in addition to numerous advantages for the surgeon. Similar patient benefits are noted with robotics as it has been shown with the use of laparoscopy for cervical, endometrial and colorectal cancer patients [6, 7, 20, 24, 31, 39-42]. However, while previous reports demonstrated longer operating times for laparoscopy, the mean operating times for robotics and laparotomy were similar in our hands, and significantly shorter as compared to laparoscopy [20]. In addition, as compared to laparoscopy, robotic patients undergoing the radical technique had significantly less blood loss and those having the modified radical technique had a significantly shorter hospitalization.

A phase III randomized clinical trial comparing laparoscopic or robotic radical hysterectomy (TLRH/TRRH) with abdominal radical hysterectomy (TARH) in patients with early stage cervical cancer is currently being performed. The aim of the study is to show the equivalence of the laparoscopic or robotic approach versus the abdominal one following a 2-phase protocol.

Robotic-Radical-Parametrectomy. Traditionally radical parametrectomy has been performed by laparotomy, with a few reports describing a vaginal laparoscopic-assisted or a total laparoscopic approach [43-45]. Ramirez *et al.*, reported the first 5 patients treated by robotic radical parametrectomy and pelvic lymphadenectomy [46]. The median operative time was 365 minutes, the estimated blood loss was 100 ml, the median number of pelvic lymph nodes was 14, and there were no conversion to laparotomy. There was one intra-operative cystotomy and one patient experienced two post-operative complications, a vesicovaginal fistula and a lymphocyst. The authors concluded that robotic radical parametrectomy and bilateral pelvic lymphadenectomy were feasible and safe with an acceptable complication rate.

Robotic Radical Trachelectomy

Vaginal radical trachelectomy in conjunction with laparoscopic pelvic lymphadenectomy to preserve fertility in women with early cervical cancer is now well established and considered to be as safe as traditional radical hysterectomy when strict selection criteria are met [47-50]. Few cases of various extent of laparoscopy in conjunction with a final vaginal approach and one case of total laparoscopic radical trachelectomy have been described [51-54]. The first report of a robotic radical trachelectomy for fertility sparing in stage IB1 adenocarcinoma of the cervix was published by Persson *et al.*, including two nulliparous women with early stage cervical cancer [55]. The long operative times of 387 and 358 minutes respectively were due to the novelty of the procedure and the required waiting time for the frozen section. No perioperative complications were observed. Their conclusion was that robotic radical trachelectomy was a safe and feasible alternative to a combined laparoscopic and vaginal approach.

Geisler *et al.*, reported a patient with a stage IB1 adenosarcoma of the cervix undergoing a robotic radical trachelectomy. The operating time was 172 minutes and the blood loss was 100 ml [56]. Burnett reported on 6 patients who underwent robotic radical trachelectomy with bilateral pelvic lymphadenectomy [57]. The authors concluded that the improved visualization and fine dissection permissible with the robotic instrumentation facilitated this operation

Ramirez PT *et al.*, published a retrospective review of all patients who underwent robotic radical trachelectomy and bilateral pelvic lymphadenectomy from October 2008 to May 2009 [58]. Included were 4 patients with early-stage squamous cell carcinoma of the cervix, 3 with stage IA2 adenocarcinoma; and 1 with stage IA1 adenocarcinoma with lymph-vascular space invasion. The median operative time was 339.5 min (range, 245 to 416). The median console time was 282.5 min (range, 217 to 338). The median estimated blood loss was 62.5 ml (range, 50 to 75). There were no conversions to laparotomy. There were no intraoperative complications. No patient required blood transfusion. The median length of hospital stay was 1.5 days (range, 1 to 2). No patient had residual tumor in the trachelectomy specimen, and no patient underwent adjuvant therapy. The median number of pelvic lymph nodes removed was 20 (range, 18 to 27).

Robotic radical trachelectomy and bilateral pelvic lymphadenectomy appear feasible and safe, and should be considered for selected patients with early cervical cancer desiring fertility-sparing surgery.

ADVANCED CERVICAL CANCER

Retroperitoneal Nodal Dissection, Transperitoneal and Extraperitoneal

Laparoscopic pelvic and paraaortic lymph node staging is widely used in patients with advanced cervical cancer prior to initiation of primary chemo-radiation therapy due to lack of sensitivity of imaging techniques. This approach has been shown to be feasible and safe [59-61]. An extended pelvic and para-aortic lymphadenectomy can be reliably and safely performed robotically in the management of gynecological malignancies. The robotic system aids in performing a meticulous dissection and in adhering to sound oncologic principles. For the robotic approach data are available for both pelvic and para-aortic lymphadenectomy performed during staging procedures for endometrial, cervical and ovarian cancers [12, 20, 30-38].

The Mayo experience on the development of a technique of robotic transperitoneal infrarenal aortic lymphadenectomy in female cadavers and the results in 33 patients who underwent the newly developed technique as part of the surgical treatment of gynecologic malignancies [62]. The mean console time was 42 minutes (range, 19-64 minutes). The mean number of nodes was 12.9 (range, 2-27); the mean number of positive nodes was 2.6 (range, 0-8). There was 1 conversion to laparotomy. The authors concluded that robotic transperitoneal infrarenal aortic lymphadenectomy can be performed adequately and safely with the robotic column at the patient's head. Operating table rotation and additional trocar sites are needed when used in conjunction with robotic pelvic surgery.

Extraperitoneal para-aortic laparoscopic lymphadenectomy is preferable to reduce the risk of adhesions prior to chemoradiation treatments and for obese patients where the transperitoneal approach can be more difficult or impossible. Data are available for the laparoscopic approach, both in terms of safety and feasibility [63-66]. Recently Vergote *et al.*, reported on 5 patients with stage IIb-IIIb cervical carcinoma who underwent robotic extraperitoneal inframesenteric para-aortic lymphadenectomy [67]. The reported results of the Leuven University series are excellent with brief hospital stays and minimal blood loss. All the procedures were completed with less than 1-hour console time. The authors concluded the robotic procedure was technically easier than the laparoscopic approach [67].

At Mayo Clinic Arizona a robotic extraperitoneal infrarenal aortic lymphadenectomy technique was developed in fresh-frozen cadavers and the resulting technique was successfully applied to a patient with cervical cancer stage IB2 presenting with enlarged aortic nodes [68]. Appropriate sites for trocar and robotic column placement were identified in the female cadavers. Docking the robot on the patient's left side gives good exposure and more freedom of movement than the traditional docking from between the legs. The operating, docking, and console times were 103, 3.5, and 49 minutes, respectively. The blood loss was 30 ml. Selective removals of 5 enlarged aortic nodes revealed no evidence of metastases. The authors concluded that robotic extraperitoneal aortic lymphadenectomy was feasible provided there is proper robotic trocar and column placement. The operating time and number of aortic nodes selectively removed by robotics in this patient are within the range of those reported with an extraperitoneal systematic aortic lymphadenectomy by laparoscopy.

RECURRENT CERVICAL CANCER

Robotic Pelvic Exenteration

Treatment of patients with recurrent cervical carcinoma after initial primary surgery or chemoradiation is based on a single or combination of treatment modalities such as radiotherapy, chemotherapy and various surgical procedures [62, 69]. Minimally invasive surgery may improve the outcome of patients with bulky residual tumor after chemoradiation due to locally advanced cervical cancer and for lateral pelvic wall recurrence. In case of central pelvic recurrence after surgery and adjuvant radiation treatment pelvic exenteration is the only therapeutic approach with curative goals. Women facing an exenterative procedure should undergo a comprehensive evaluation to make sure there is no evidence of unresectable or metastatic disease that would make them unsuitable candidates for exenteration. The laparoscopic approach for a pre-treatment evaluation in patients with recurrent cervical cancer has already shown to be paramount to select adequate candidates for exenterative procedure similarly a pre-exenteration robotic evaluation can be easily performed [70, 71].

Pruthi *et al.*, recently described the technique of robotic-assisted anterior pelvic exenteration performed in 12 women for clinically localized bladder cancer [72]. Nine patients underwent ileal conduit diversion and three patients underwent an orthotopic neobladder. In all cases, the urinary diversion was performed extracorporeally. Mean operating room time was 4.6 hours; mean surgical blood loss was 221 ml. Mean time to flatus was 1.9 days and to bowel movement 2.4 days, and time to discharge 4.8 days. There were two postoperative complications (17%) in two patients. The authors' initial experience with robotic-assisted laparoscopic anterior pelvic exenteration appears to be favorable with acceptable operative, pathologic, and short-term clinical outcomes. However, the oncological outcomes of these new minimally invasive surgical approaches need to be carefully verified through larger experiences to adequately evaluate and validate these procedures as appropriate surgical and oncologic options.

OVARIAN CANCER

Early Ovarian Cancer

Most cases of ovarian cancer are diagnosed as advanced stages, the few that are diagnosed as early stages need a staging procedure. Staging procedure for an apparent early ovarian cancer includes total hysterectomy bilateral salpingo-oophorectomy, pelvic and peri-aortic lymphadenectomy, and omentectomy and these procedures can be performed using a minimally invasive approach.

Prospective trials and retrospective analyses have demonstrated the safety and feasibility of laparoscopy in performing hysterectomy, bilateral salpingo-oophorectomy, and pelvic and periaortic lymphadenectomy for surgical staging [12-19, 73]. The use of minimally invasive techniques does not appear to have an adverse impact on survival, and it improves quality of life in the postoperative period. However, the learning curve for the laparoscopic approach has been shown to be difficult and long, in particular when the goal is infrarenal periaortic lymphadenectomy.

Advanced and Recurrent Ovarian Cancer

Primary maximal surgical effort is currently considered standard of care in newly diagnosed ovarian cancer patients. Unfortunately, numerous studies have shown that many women with ovarian cancer do not undergo optimal surgery and limitations, however, have been postulated to this treatment strategy. First, patients with residual disease larger than 2 cm have no meaningful impact on overall survival [74]. Second, an acceptable optimal primary cytoreduction rate defined as residual tumor less than 1 cm is most likely obtained by specialized surgeons, gynecologic oncologists with extended formal training in cytoreductive techniques [75-77]. Unfortunately, there seems to be a scarce access for the overall population of women with ovarian cancer to a specialized gynecologist and institutions. Consequently, alternative strategies such as neoadjuvant chemotherapy (NACT) for up-front treatment of newly diagnosed ovarian cancer patients have been proposed [78].

Robotic surgery for more advanced ovarian cancer with carcinomatosis is challenging because of the need to operate in all four quadrants of the abdomen therefore in this setting neoadjuvant chemotherapy could have a role. In the authors' experience, the ability to operate in all four quadrants can best be achieved by rotating the operating table and redocking the robot at the patient's head. In this position, as mentioned earlier, it is possible to excise paraaortic lymph nodes to the level of the renal vessels and to perform resection of upper abdominal metastases. This position also allows for debulking of diaphragm metastases and or involving the liver. In such setting the robotic system is helpful in avoiding the need for extensive mobilization of the liver needed to perform similar diaphragm debulking through laparotomy. Finally, the reverse-docking position is helpful when the transverse colon needs to be mobilized for bowel resection.

Data on the application of robotic technology for advanced ovarian cancer is scant. There are only case reports or series in the literature that document the experience with ovarian carcinoma and robotic-assisted laparoscopy with no subgroup analysis specifically for patients with ovarian cancer [79-82]. Mean operating time and blood loss were not specifically reported for the subset of patients with ovarian cancer. Van Dam *et al.*, reported on a patient with breast lobular carcinoma that had metastasized to the ovaries [83]. The patient was successfully treated with robotic-assisted debulking surgery involving bilateral salpingo-oophorectomy. The procedure time was 200 minutes, blood loss was 300 mL, and there were no intraoperative or postoperative complications.

Bandera reported that between January 2006 and February 2008, the group at Mayo Hospital Phoenix performed 21 robotic surgeries for ovarian cancer including 12 primary debulking/staging procedures, four interval debulking procedures following neoadjuvant chemotherapy, and five secondary debulking procedures [84]. In addition to hysterectomy, bilateral salpingo-oophorectomy, omentectomy, and lymphadenectomy, several radical procedures were performed using the robot such as modified pelvic exenteration with rectosigmoid resection, small bowel resection, diaphragm resection, and hepatic metastases resection. Operative times for these procedures ranged from 103 to 454 min, and estimated blood loss ranged from 0 to 300 ml. Perioperative complications were minimal. The authors concluded that based on their experience robotic surgery may play a role in the treatment of carefully selected patients with advanced ovarian cancer, but there exist a few disadvantages in the implementation of robotic-assisted surgery for ovarian cancer such as the need for table rotation, increased number of trocars, increased operating time with increased number of procedures and the need for abdominal incision for anastomosis or removal of large specimens.

The use of the surgical robotic system can be also advocated in the case of isolated recurrence of ovarian cancer such as in the pelvis or in the upper abdomen on the diaphragm or metastatic to the liver. Robotic surgery for hepatic resection has not yet been extensively reported. Choi *et al.*, reported on 3 robot-assisted left lateral excision of the liver performed between March and May 2007 [85]. All procedures were successful and patients recovered without complications. Shorter lengths of hospital stay, earlier start of oral feeding and less amount of ascites were found. The authors concluded that robotic hepatic surgery is still a new field in its developing stage. In patients with small malignant tumors robotic-assisted resection is feasible and safe; however, careful patient selection is important and long-term outcomes need to be evaluated.

CONCLUSION

Robotics and conventional laparoscopy are preferable to laparotomy for suitable patients with cervical, endometrial cancer, and early ovarian cancer. Although prospective randomized trials are desirable, the present evidence strongly supports the use of MIS for endometrial and cervical cancer patients.

REFERENCES

[1]   Moorthy K, Munz Y, Dosis A, *et al.* Dexterity enhancement with robotic surgery. Surg Endosc 2004; 18(5): 790-5.
[2]   Prasad SM, Prasad SM, Maniar HS, *et al.* Surgical robotics: impact of motion scaling on task performance. J Am Coll Surg 2004; 199(6): 863-8.
[3]   Sarle R, Tewari A, Shrivastava A, Peabody J, Menon M. Surgical robotics and laparoscopic training drills. J Endourol 2004; 18(1): 63-6; discussion 6-7.
[4]   Yohannes P, Rotariu P, Pinto P, Smith AD, Lee BR. Comparison of robotic versus laparoscopic skills: is there a difference in the learning curve? Urology 2002; 60(1): 39-45; discussion
[5]   Cho YH, Kim DY, Kim JH, *et al.* Laparoscopic management of early uterine cancer: 10-year experience in Asan Medical Center. Gynecol Oncol 2007; 106(3): 585-90.
[6]   Magrina JF. Outcomes of laparoscopic treatment for endometrial cancer. Curr Opin Obstet Gynecol 2005; 17(4): 343-6.
[7]   Magrina JF, Mutone NF, Weaver AL, *et al.* Laparoscopic lymphadenectomy and vaginal or laparoscopic hysterectomy with bilateral salpingo-oophorectomy for endometrial cancer: morbidity and survival. Am J Obstet Gynecol 1999; 181(2): 376-81.
[8]   Eltabbakh GH, Shamonki MI, Moody JM, Garafano LL. Laparoscopy as the primary modality for the treatment of women with endometrial carcinoma. Cancer 2001; 91(2): 378-87.
[9]   Frumovitz M, dos Reis R, Sun CC, *et al.* Comparison of total laparoscopic and abdominal radical hysterectomy for patients with early-stage cervical cancer. Obstet Gynecol 2007; 110(1): 96-102.
[10]   Malur S, Possover M, Michels W, Schneider A. Laparoscopic-assisted vaginal versus abdominal surgery in patients with endometrial cancer--a prospective randomized trial. Gynecol Oncol 2001; 80(2): 239-44.
[11]   Zakashansky K, Chuang L, Gretz H, *et al.* A case-controlled study of total laparoscopic radical hysterectomy with pelvic lymphadenectomy versus radical abdominal hysterectomy in a fellowship training program. Int J Gynecol Cancer 2007; 17(5): 1075-82.
[12]   DeNardis SA, Holloway RW, Bigsby GEt, *et al.* Robotically assisted laparoscopic hysterectomy versus total abdominal hysterectomy and lymphadenectomy for endometrial cancer. Gynecol Oncol 2008; 111(3): 412-7.
[13]   Peiretti M, Zanagnolo V, Bocciolone L, *et al.* Robotic surgery: changing the surgical approach for endometrial cancer in a referral cancer center. J Minim Invasive Gynecol 2009; 16(4): 427-31.
[14]   Veljovich DS, Paley PJ, Drescher CW, *et al.* Robotic surgery in gynecologic oncology: program initiation and outcomes after the first year with comparison with laparotomy for endometrial cancer staging. Am J Obstet Gynecol 2008; 198(6): 679 e1-9; discussion e9-10.
[15]   Bell MC, Torgerson J, Seshadri-Kreaden U, Suttle AW, Hunt S. Comparison of outcomes and cost for endometrial cancer staging *via* traditional laparotomy, standard laparoscopy and robotic techniques. Gynecol Oncol 2008; 111(3): 407-11.
[16]   Boggess JF, Gehrig PA, Cantrell L, *et al.* A comparative study of 3 surgical methods for hysterectomy with staging for endometrial cancer: robotic assistance, laparoscopy, laparotomy. Am J Obstet Gynecol 2008; 199(4): 360 e1-9.

[17]   Gehrig PA, Cantrell LA, Shafer A, *et al.* What is the optimal minimally invasive surgical procedure for endometrial cancer staging in the obese and morbidly obese woman? Gynecol Oncol 2008; 111(1): 41-5.

[18]   Holloway RW, Ahmad S, DeNardis SA, *et al.* Robotic-assisted laparoscopic hysterectomy and lymphadenectomy for endometrial cancer: Analysis of surgical performance. Gynecol Oncol 2009; 115(3): 447-52.

[19]   Seamon LG, Cohn DE, Henretta MS, *et al.* Minimally invasive comprehensive surgical staging for endometrial cancer: Robotics or laparoscopy? Gynecol Oncol 2009; 113(1): 36-41.

[20]   Magrina JF, Kho RM, Weaver AL, Montero RP, Magtibay PM. Robotic radical hysterectomy: comparison with laparoscopy and laparotomy. Gynecol Onco 2008; 109(1): 86-91.

[21]   Zullo F, Palomba S, Russo T, *et al.* A prospective randomized comparison between laparoscopic and laparotomic approaches in women with early stage endometrial cancer: a focus on the quality of life. Am J Obstet Gynecol 2005; 193(4): 1344-52.

[22]   Noel JK, Fahrbach K, Estok R, *et al.* Minimally invasive colorectal resection outcomes: short-term comparison with open procedures. J Am Coll Surg 2007; 204(2): 291-307.

[23]   Visco AG, Advincula AP. Robotic gynecologic surgery. Obstet Gynecol 2008; 112(6): 1369-84.

[24]   Holloway RW, Finkler NJ, Pikaart DP, *et al.* Comparison of total laparoscopic and abdominal radical hysterectomy for patients with early-stage cervical cancer. Obstet Gynecol 2007; 110(5): 1174; author reply -5.

[25]   Magrina JF. Robotic surgery in gynecology. Eur J Gynaecol Oncol 2007; 28(2): 77-82.

[26]   Puntambekar SP, Palep RJ, Puntambekar SS, *et al.* Laparoscopic total radical hysterectomy by the Pune technique: our experience of 248 cases. J Minim Invasive Gynecol 2007; 14(6): 682-9.

[27]   Zakashansky K, Lerner DL. Total laparoscopic radical hysterectomy for the treatment of cervical cancer. J Minim Invasive Gynecol 2008; 15(3): 387-8; author reply 8.

[28]   Obermair A, Gebski V, Frumovitz M, *et al.* A phase III randomized clinical trial comparing laparoscopic or robotic radical hysterectomy with abdominal radical hysterectomy in patients with early stage cervical cancer. J Minim Invasive Gynecol 2008; 15(5): 584-8.

[29]   Magrina JF, Kho R, Magtibay PM. Robotic radical hysterectomy: Technical aspects. Gynecol Oncol 2009; 113(1): 28-31.

[30]   Boggess JF, Gehrig PA, Cantrell L, *et al.* A case-control study of robot-assisted type III radical hysterectomy with pelvic lymph node dissection compared with open radical hysterectomy. Am J Obstet Gynecol 2008; 199(4): 357 e1-7.

[31]   Estape R, Lambrou N, Diaz R, *et al.* A case matched analysis of robotic radical hysterectomy with lymphadenectomy compared with laparoscopy and laparotomy. Gynecol Oncol 2009; 113(3): 357-61.

[32]   Fanning J, Fenton B, Purohit M. Robotic radical hysterectomy. Am J Obstet Gynecol 2008; 198(6): 649 e1-4.

[33]   Kim YT, Kim SW, Hyung WJ, *et al.* Robotic radical hysterectomy with pelvic lymphadenectomy for cervical carcinoma: a pilot study. Gynecol Oncol 2008; 108(2): 312-6.

[34]   Maggioni A, Minig L, Zanagnolo V, *et al.* Robotic approach for cervical cancer: comparison with laparotomy: a case control study. Gynecol Oncol 2009; 115(1): 60-4.

[35]   Nezhat FR, Datta MS, Liu C, Chuang L, Zakashansky K. Robotic radical hysterectomy versus total laparoscopic radical hysterectomy with pelvic lymphadenectomy for treatment of early cervical cancer. JSLS 2008; 12(3): 227-37.

[36]   Persson J, Reynisson P, Borgfeldt C, *et al.* Robot assisted laparoscopic radical hysterectomy and pelvic lymphadenectomy with short and long term morbidity data. Gynecol Oncol 2009 May; 113(2):185-90.

[37]   Sert BM, Abeler VM. Robotic-assisted laparoscopic radical hysterectomy (Piver type III) with pelvic node dissection-- case report. Eur J Gynaecol Oncol 2006; 27(5): 531-3.

[38]   Sert B, Abeler V. Robotic radical hysterectomy in early-stage cervical carcinoma patients, comparing results with total laparoscopic radical hysterectomy cases. The future is now? Int J Med Robot 2007; 3(3): 224-8.

[39]   Hewett PJ, Allardyce RA, Bagshaw PF, *et al.* Short-term outcomes of the Australasian randomized clinical study comparing laparoscopic and conventional open surgical treatments for colon cancer: the ALCCaS trial. Ann Surg 2008; 248(5): 728-38.

[40]   Kehoe SM, Ramirez PT, Abu-Rustum NR. Innovative laparoscopic surgery in gynecologic oncology. Curr Oncol Rep 2007; 9(6): 472-7.

[41]   Magrina JF, Weaver AL. Laparoscopic treatment of endometrial cancer: five-year recurrence and survival rates. Eur J Gynaecol Oncol 2004; 25(4): 439-41.

[42]   Nezhat F, Yadav J, Rahaman J, Gretz H, Cohen C. Analysis of survival after laparoscopic management of endometrial cancer. J Minim Invasive Gynecol 2008; 15(2): 181-7.

[43]   Lee CL, Huang KG. Total laparoscopic radical parametrectomy. J Minim Invasive Gynecol 2005; 12(2): 168-70.

[44]   Liang Z, Xu H, Chen Y, *et al.* Laparoscopic radical trachelectomy or parametrectomy and pelvic and para-aortic lymphadenectomy for cervical or vaginal stump carcinoma: report of six cases. Int J Gynecol Cancer 2006; 16(4): 1713-6.

[45] Nezhat F, Prasad Hayes M, Peiretti M, Rahaman J. Laparoscopic radical parametrectomy and partial vaginectomy for recurrent endometrial cancer. Gynecol Oncol 2007; 104(2): 494-6.

[46] Ramirez PT, Schmeler KM, Wolf JK, Brown J, Soliman PT. Robotic radical parametrectomy and pelvic lymphadenectomy in patients with invasive cervical cancer. Gynecol Oncol 2008; 111(1): 18-21.

[47] Beiner ME, Hauspy J, Rosen B, et al. Radical vaginal trachelectomy vs. radical hysterectomy for small early stage cervical cancer: a matched case-control study. Gynecol Oncol 2008; 110(2): 168-71.

[48] Diaz JP, Sonoda Y, Leitao MM, et al. Oncologic outcome of fertility-sparing radical trachelectomy versus radical hysterectomy for stage IB1 cervical carcinoma. Gynecol Oncol 2008; 111(2): 255-60.

[49] Einstein MH, Park KJ, Sonoda Y, et al. Radical vaginal versus abdominal trachelectomy for stage IB1 cervical cancer: a comparison of surgical and pathologic outcomes. Gynecol Oncol 2009; 112(1): 73-7.

[50] Shepherd JH, Spencer C, Herod J, Ind TE. Radical vaginal trachelectomy as a fertility-sparing procedure in women with early-stage cervical cancer-cumulative pregnancy rate in a series of 123 women. Bjog 2006; 113(6): 719-24.

[51] Chen Y, Xu H, Zhang Q, et al. A fertility-preserving option in early cervical carcinoma: laparoscopy-assisted vaginal radical trachelectomy and pelvic lymphadenectomy. Eur J Obstet Gynecol Reprod Biol 2008; 136(1): 90-3.

[52] Diaz-Feijoo B, Gil-Moreno A, Puig O, Martinez-Palones JM, Xercavins J. Total laparoscopic radical trachelectomy with intraoperative sentinel node identification for early cervical stump cancer. J Minim Invasive Gynecol. 2005; 12(6): 522-4.

[53] Gorchev G, Tomov S. [Laparoscopically assisted radical vaginal trachelectomy--first attempt]. Akush Ginekol (Sofiia) 2005; 44(7): 56-60.

[54] Marchiole P, Benchaib M, Buenerd A, et al. Oncological safety of laparoscopic-assisted vaginal radical trachelectomy (LARVT or Dargent's operation): a comparative study with laparoscopic-assisted vaginal radical hysterectomy (LARVH). Gynecol Oncol 2007; 106(1): 132-41.

[55] Persson J, Kannisto P, Bossmar T. Robot-assisted abdominal laparoscopic radical trachelectomy. Gynecol Oncol 2008; 111(3): 564-7.

[56] Geisler JP, Orr CJ, Manahan KJ. Robotically assisted total laparoscopic radical trachelectomy for fertility sparing in stage IB1 adenosarcoma of the cervix. J Laparoendosc Adv Surg Tech A 2008; 18(5): 727-9.

[57] Burnett AF, Stone PJ, Duckworth LA, Roman JJ. Robotic radical trachelectomy for preservation of fertility in early cervical cancer: case series and description of technique. J Minim Invasive Gynecol 2009; 16(5): 569-72.

[58] Ramirez PT, Schmeler KM, Malpica A, Soliman PT. Safety and feasibility of robotic radical trachelectomy in patients with early-stage cervical cancer. Gynecol Oncol 2010; 116(3): 512-5.

[59] Kehoe SM, Abu-Rustum NR. Transperitoneal laparoscopic pelvic and paraaortic lymphadenectomy in gynecologic cancers. Curr Treat Options Oncol 2006; 7(2): 93-101.

[60] Marnitz S, Kohler C, Roth C, et al. Is there a benefit of pretreatment laparoscopic transperitoneal surgical staging in patients with advanced cervical cancer? Gynecol Oncol. 2005 Dec;99(3):536-44.

[61] Papadia A, Remorgida V, Salom EM, Ragni N. Laparoscopic pelvic and paraaortic lymphadenectomy in gynecologic oncology. J Am Assoc Gynecol Laparosc 2004; 11(3): 297-306.

[62] Magrina JF, Long JB, Kho RM, et al. Robotic transperitoneal infrarenal aortic lymphadenectomy: technique and results. Int J Gynecol Cancer 2010; 20(1): 184-7.

[63] Burnett AF, O'Meara AT, Bahador A, Roman LD, Morrow CP. Extraperitoneal laparoscopic lymph node staging: the University of Southern California experience. Gynecol Oncol 2004; 95(1): 189-92.

[64] Gil-Moreno A, Franco-Camps S, Diaz-Feijoo B, et al. Usefulness of extraperitoneal laparoscopic paraaortic lymphadenectomy for lymph node recurrence in gynecologic malignancy. Acta Obstet Gynecol Scand 2008; 87(7): 723-30.

[65] Querleu D, Dargent D, Ansquer Y, Leblanc E, Narducci F. Extraperitoneal endosurgical aortic and common iliac dissection in the staging of bulky or advanced cervical carcinomas. Cancer 2000; 88(8): 1883-91.

[66] Tillmanns T, Lowe MP. Safety, feasibility, and costs of outpatient laparoscopic extraperitoneal aortic nodal dissection for locally advanced cervical carcinoma. Gynecol Oncol 2007; 106(2): 370-4.

[67] Vergote I, Pouseele B, Van Gorp T, et al. Robotic retroperitoneal lower para-aortic lymphadenectomy in cervical carcinoma: first report on the technique used in 5 patients. Acta Obstet Gynecol Scand 2008; 87(7): 783-7.

[68] Elst P, Ahankour F, Tjalma W. Management of recurrent cervical cancer. Review of the literature and case report. Eur J Gynaecol Oncol. 2007;28(6):435-41.

[69] Chiva LM, Lapuente F, Gonzalez-Cortijo L, et al. Surgical treatment of recurrent cervical cancer: state of the art and new achievements. Gynecol Oncol 2008; 110(3 Suppl 2): S60-6.

[70] Leblanc F, Narducci F, Chevalier A, et al. Pretherapeutic laparoscopic staging of locally advanced cervical carcinomas: technique and results. Gynecol Oncol 2005; 99(3 Suppl 1): S157-8.

[71] Pectasides D, Kamposioras K, Papaxoinis G, Pectasides E. Chemotherapy for recurrent cervical cancer. Cancer Treat Rev 2008; 34(7): 603-13.

[72] Pruthi RS, Stefaniak H, Hubbard JS, Wallen EM. Robot-assisted laparoscopic anterior pelvic exenteration for bladder cancer in the female patient. J Endourol 2008; 22(10): 2397-402; discussion 402.

[73] Humphrey MM, Apte SM. The use of minimally invasive surgery for endometrial cancer. Cancer Control 2009; 16(1): 30-7.

[74] Hoskins WJ. Epithelial ovarian carcinoma: principles of primary surgery. Gynecol Oncol 1994; 55(3 Pt 2): S91-6.

[75] Bristow RE, Tomacruz RS, Armstrong DK, Trimble EL, Montz FJ. Survival effect of maximal cytoreductive surgery for advanced ovarian carcinoma during the platinum era: a meta-analysis. J Clin Oncol 2002; 20(5): 1248-59.

[76] Eisenkop SM, Friedman RL, Wang HJ. Complete cytoreductive surgery is feasible and maximizes survival in patients with advanced epithelial ovarian cancer: a prospective study. Gynecol Oncol 1998 May;69(2):103-8.

[77] Vernooij F, Heintz P, Witteveen E, van der Graaf Y. The outcomes of ovarian cancer treatment are better when provided by gynecologic oncologists and in specialized hospitals: a systematic review. Gynecol Oncol 2007 Jun;105(3): 801-12.

[78] Vergote I, De Wever I, Tjalma W, *et al.* Neoadjuvant chemotherapy or primary debulking surgery in advanced ovarian carcinoma: a retrospective analysis of 285 patients. Gynecol Oncol 1998; 71(3): 431-6.

[79] Diaz-Arrastia C, Jurnalov C, Gomez G, Townsend C, Jr. Laparoscopic hysterectomy using a computer-enhanced surgical robot. Surg Endosc 2002; 16(9): 1271-3.

[80] Field JB, Benoit MF, Dinh TA, Diaz-Arrastia C. Computer-enhanced robotic surgery in gynecologic oncology. Surg Endosc 2007; 21(2): 244-6.

[81] Kho RM, Hilger WS, Hentz JG, Magtibay PM, Magrina JF. Robotic hysterectomy: technique and initial outcomes. Am J Obstet Gynecol 2007; 197(1): 113 e1-4.

[82] Lambaudie E, Houvenaeghel G, Walz J, *et al.* Robot-assisted laparoscopy in gynecologic oncology. Surg Endosc 2008; 22(12): 2743-7.

[83] van Dam PA, van Dam PJ, Verkinderen L, *et al.* Robotic-assisted laparoscopic cytoreductive surgery for lobular carcinoma of the breast metastatic to the ovaries. J Minim Invasive Gynecol 2007; 14(6): 746-9.

[84] Bandera CA, Magrina JF. Robotic surgery in gynecologic oncology. Curr Opin Obstet Gynecol 2009; 21(1): 25-30.

[85] Choi SB, Park JS, Kim JK, *et al.* Early experiences of robotic-assisted laparoscopic liver resection. Yonsei Med J 2008; 49(4): 632-8

CHAPTER 7

Complications of Gynecologic Robotic Surgery

Geetu Pahlajani and Tommaso Falcone*

Professor and Chair Obstetrics, Gynecology and Women's Health Institute, Cleveland Clinic, 9500 Euclid Ave - A81, Cleveland, Ohio USA

Abstract: Robotic technology represents a significant advancement in the field of minimal invasive surgery. Robotic procedures are increasingly used to perform various gynecological operations. While the robot addresses the limitations of the laparoscope and provides three-dimensional vision and precise movements, it has its some limitations including increased cost, bulky instrument with limited vaginal access, and lack of tactile feedback. Although the literature has shown that robotic surgery leads to early recovery and less blood loss, it is associated with increased operative time, which is associated with potential increase of anesthetic and perioperative complications. This article reviews the recent peer-reviewed literature concerning the complications of robotic technology in hysterectomy, myomectomy, tubal anastomosis, and sacrocolpopexy. Most of the literature consists of retrospective studies and authors' early experiences with this technique. Well designed prospective studies are necessary to determine the long-term outcomes including complications.

INTRODUCTION

Over the past few decades minimal invasive procedures have been extensively performed for various gynecological disorders, including gynecological cancers. Substantial decrease in the length of hospital stay, decreased need for postoperative analgesia and improved recovery time have made this surgical approach popular amongst the surgeons and the patients. However, the conventional laparoscope has some limitations such as limited mobility of straight instruments, two-dimensional imaging, poor ergonomic position for the surgeon and a steep learning curve.

Robotic platform addresses these limitations and offers several advantages over laparoscopy including wristed instrumentation, three dimensional vision system, and ergonomic positioning of the surgeon. These advantages offer familiar environment similar to that of laparotomy approach, greater degree of mobility and technical ease for the surgeon. However, it is associated with certain complications. In this article we will address the limitations and complications associated with the robotic surgery in gynecological practice.

LIMITATIONS OF ROBOTIC SURGERY IN GYNECOLOGY

One of the main limitations of robotic assisted surgery is the high cost. The cost to install the da Vinci robotic platform is approximately $1.5 million with a 10% annual maintenance fee. Additional costs include training of surgeons and the operating room personnel and increased operative time for robotic setup and docking. Chung *et al* did a cost effective analysis for hysterectomy using laparotomy, laparoscopy and robotic associated laparoscopy and found the laparoscopic approach to be most cost effective [1]. However, cost analysis study in urological and cardiology robotic surgery demonstrated that after the initial investment and once the learning curve has been overcome, robotic assisted surgery becomes cost-effective [2].

The amount of case volume in a given institution needs to be taken under consideration before the economic benefits are analyzed. Currently, it appears that robotic technology is most cost-effective in settings of high case volume. Another limitation is the learning curve associated with the robotic surgeries, which adds to the cost of the technology. Lenihan *et al* evaluated robotically assisted laparoscopic surgeries for benign gynecological disorders and concluded that it took about 50 cases to stabilize the operative time [3]. In another series, Seamon *et al* demonstrated that the learning curve for endometrial cancer staging using the robotic technology required only 20 cases to reach the state of efficiency [4]. The learning curve for robotic surgeries seems to be smaller if not at par to the laparoscopic surgery [5,6]. Studies comparing the learning curve of these two techniques have never been performed. Similar to other surgical techniques, the proficiency of robotic surgeries improves over time.

*Address correspondence to Tommaso Falcone: Professor and Chair Obstetrics, Gynecology and Women's Health Institute, Cleveland Clinic, 9500 Euclid Ave - A81, Cleveland, Ohio USA, 44195: Tel: [216]444-1758; Fax: [216]445-6325; Email: falcont@ccf.org

Lack of tactile feedback is a drawback associated with the robots. The depth of perception through the three-dimensional vision compensates for this limitation for most surgeons over time. Another downside is the limited vaginal access after the robot has been docked. For example, it is more difficult to use a uterine manipulator during robotic surgery than at conventional laparoscopy. The side docking technique overcomes this limitation.

Another disadvantage of robotic assisted operation is the need for larger incisions [>8mm] than that for a conventional laparoscopic surgery. Although trocar site herniation is a rare complication of laparoscopic surgery with smaller than 10mm size ports [7], Seamon *et al* reported a case of small bowel evisceration through an 8mm robotic port after endometrial cancer staging surgery [8]. Inability to operate in both the upper and lower abdomen simultaneously during gynecological cancer surgeries is another limitation of robotic surgery. The robot must be undocked after a pelvic surgery and redocked again facing the upper abdomen for the aortic lymph node dissection which adds to the duration of the anesthesia and surgery.

COMPLICATION OF ROBOTIC ASSISTED HYSTERECTOMY

Hysterectomy is one of the most common gynecological operations performed either by abdominal, vaginal or laparoscopic route [9]. Minimal invasive techniques lead to reduced blood loss, early recovery, and short hospital stay and has gained popularity amongst the patients. However, it is associated with long operative time, increased incidence of urinary tract injuries and a steep learning curve [10]. Robotic surgery has been advocated as a possible way to circumvent these limitations.

Several authors have reported their experiences with robotic hysterectomy (Table **1**). They reported complications such as occasional cases of visceral injury, vaginal laceration, vaginal cuff bleeding or abscess, and vaginal cuff separation (Table **2**). Payne *et al* compared the surgical outcomes of robotic assisted hysterectomy to total laparoscopic hysterectomy. They concluded that robotic hysterectomy was quicker with less blood loss and reduced risk of abdominal conversion than a standard laparoscopy [11]. In another study, Shashoua *et al* compared robotic assisted total laparoscopic hysterectomy and conventional total laparoscopic hysterectomy. Although they found improved post-operative recovery in robotic surgery, they encountered challenges with operating large uterus. In addition, they had a difficulty to remove a large uterus vaginally due to poor visualization for morcellation by the vaginal route. This required undocking the robot for the safe removal of the specimen [12]. Side docking might overcome this limitation.

Table 1: Published cases of robotic hysterectomy

Authors	Beste, *et al* [18]	Fiorentino, *et al* [19]	Reynolds & Advincula [20]	Kho, *et al* [21]	Payne & Dauterive [11]	Lenihan, *et al* [22]	Boggers, *et al* [23]	Nezhat, *et al* [24]
Patients [n]	11	20	16	91	100	113	152	26
BMI [kg/m2]	26.0	NR	27.8	27.9	28.8	29.0	30.7	25.4
Uterine weight [g]	49-227	98	132	136	267	184	347	255
Operative time [min]	192	200	242	128	119	107	122.9	276
EBL [ml]	25-350	81	96	79	61	103	79.0	250
Conversion rate [%]	9.1	10.0	0	0	4.0	1.8	0	0
LOS [days]	1.0	2.0	1.5	1.35	1.1	1.0	1.0	1.0
Complication rate [%]	0	5.0	25.0	6.6	2.0	3.5	5.2	0

Results are presented as mean, number [n] and percentages [%]. BMI= body mass index, EBL= estimated blood loss, LOS= length of stay, NR=not reported, Complications up to 6 weeks post-operatively.

Table 2: Reported complications after robotic hysterectomy.

Authors	Beste, et al [18]	Fiorentino, et al [19]	Reynolds & Advincula [20]	Kho, et al [21]	Payne & Dauterive [11]	Lenihan, et al [22]	Boggers, et al [23]	Nezhat, et al [24]
No. patients	11	20	16	91	100	113	152	26
Pneumonia	0	0	1 [6.25%]	1 [1.1%]	0	0	0	0
Post-op infection	0	0	1	0	0	1 [0.88%]	3 [1.97%]	0
Vaginal cuff abscess/hematoma	0	1 [5%]	1 [6.25%]	1 [1.1%]	1 [1%]	0	2 [1.32%]	0
Vaginal cuff dehiscence	0	0	0	0	0	1 [0.88%]	0	0
Bowel injury	0	0	1 [6.25%]	0	0	0	1 [0.66%]	0
Ureteral/bladder injury	0	0	0	0	1 [1%]	1 [0.88%]	1 [0.66%]	0
Vaginal laceration	0	0	0	0	0	1 [0.88%]	1 [0.66%]	0
Others	0	0	0	4 [4.4%]	0	0	0	0

Payne *et al* published their experience with robotically assisted hysterectomy in patients with large uterus and concluded that robotic hysterectomy was associated with less morbidity and blood loss. The overall complication rate was 3.5%; this included vaginal cuff infections, cuff dehiscence and cystotomies [13]. Kho *et al* reported a 4.1% incidence of vaginal cuff dehiscence after robotic hysterectomy. They attributed this complication to thermal injury and to the vaginal closure technique [14]. It appears that vaginal cuff dehiscence may occur more often after conventional laparoscopic hysterectomy [1.1%] than after other hysterectomy approaches [15]. The higher rate with robotic hysterectomy may be related to the technique of laparoscopic suturing.

Another complication that might be unique to robotic assisted hysterectomy is a lower limb compartment syndrome. This could be related to the prolonged operative time. For example the mean operative time for robotic hysterectomy in patients with endometrial cancer ranges from 177 to 283 minutes [16], and the chances of developing a lower limb compartment syndrome increase in long duration multidisciplinary surgeries. Tomassetti reported a case of lower limb compartment syndrome during a prolonged laparoscopic surgery for extensive endometriosis [17]. Appropriate measures should be taken during robotic surgeries to prevent this complication.

COMPLICATION OF ROBOTIC-ASSISTED MYOMECTOMY

Compared to myomectomy by laparotomy, laparoscopic myomectomy is associated with rapid post-operative recovery, shorter hospital stay, and less adhesion formation [25]. However, laparoscopic myomectomy is a demanding technique requiring multilayered closure of the uterine defect. As a result, it may lead to conversion to laparotomy. Robotic-assisted myomectomy provides advanced imaging, improved instrument dexterity and precision, and better-targeted coagulation.

In a retrospective study, Advincula *et al* compared robotic-assisted myomectomy to myomectomy by laparotomy. They reported longer operative time with the use of robot as well as a case of cardiogenic shock due to vasopressin. No intraoperative complication was encountered in the laparotomy group. The postoperative complications in the laparotomy group were higher than in the robotic group [26]. Nezhat *et al* compared the robotic and the laparoscopic myomectomy. They found no major advantage of the robotic technique but confirmed the prolonged surgical time [27]. Similar results were reported by Bedient *et al.* They encountered difficulties to remove large fibroid and to obtain adequate homeostasis of a large bleeding site with robotic assisted myomectomy [28] (Tables **3** and **4**). Yet, they reported less intraoperative and postoperative complication rates with robotic myomectomy as compared to laparoscopic myomectomy.

Table 3: Published cases of myomectomy by laparotomy, by laparoscopy, and robotic assisted myomectomy.

Authors	Advincula, *et al* [26]		Nezhat, *et al* [27]		Bedient, *et al* [28]		George, *et al* [29]
Technique	Robot	Laparotomy	Robot	Laparoscopy	Robot	Laparoscopy	Robotic
Patients [n]	29	29	15	35	41	40	77
BMI [Kg/m^2]	25.3	28.3	23	24	24.7	25.3	28.1
Myoma weight [g]	227.8	223.7	116	156	210	350	235.0
Operative time [min]	231.3	154.4	234	203	141	166	195
EBL [ml]	195.6	364.6	370	420	100	250	100
Transfusion rate [%]	0	6.9	0	0	5	12.1	2.5
LOS [days]	1.4	3.6	1.0	1.05	NR	NR	1
Complication rate [%]	48.2	13.7	0	0	12.1	35	3.8

Results are presented as mean, number [n] and percentages [%]. BMI= body mass index, EBL= estimated blood loss, LOS= length of stay, NR=not reported.

Table 4: Complications of robotic assisted myomectomy.

Authors	Advincula, *et al* [26]	Nezhat, *et al* [27]	Bedient, *et al* [28]
No. of patients	29	15	41
Intra-operative Cardiogenic shock Bleeding	 1 [3.45%] 0	 0 0	 0 1 [2.44%]
Post-operative Pneumonia Chest pain Wound infection Bowel Injury Pelvic abscess Blood transfusion	 1 [3.45%] 1 [3.45%] 1 [3.45%] 0 0 0	 0 0 0 0 0 0	 1 [2.44%] 0 2 [4.88%] 1 [2.44%] 1 [2.44%] 2 [4.88%]

Recently, George *et al* studied the impact of body mass index [BMI] on the surgical outcomes of patients undergoing robotic myomectomy [29]. They encountered a difficulty in obtaining the pneumoperitoneum in the obese patients but did not report any intraoperative complications [29]. They found no evidence that increased BMI worsened the surgical outcomes.

COMPLICATION OF ROBOTIC-ASSISTED TUBAL ANASTOMOSIS

In 2000, Degueldre *et al* published their experience of robotic assisted tubal anastomosis in eight patients. They reported favorable operative time with the use of robots, but found the absence of tactile feedback as a disadvantage [30]. In their small series, the y did not encounter any complication. Rodgers *et al* compared the outcomes of tubal anastomosis by robots and open method, and found increased operative time and shorter recovery time with the use of robots. They encountered one postoperative tachycardia in the robotic group and complications among 6 cases in the laparotomy group [31]. Patel *et al*, prospectively compared robotic to open microsurgical tubal anastomosis, and confirmed the increased operative time with robotic surgery. There was one case of trocar injury to the epigastric artery in the robotic group. Pregnancy rates were comparable in the two groups, yet the robotic group had a higher numbers of ectopic pregnancies (Table **5**) [32].

Table 5: Tubal anastomosis with or without robotic assistance.

Authors	Falcone, *et al* [31]		Patel, *et al* [32]	
Technique	Robotic	Open	Robotic	Open
No. patients	26	41	18	10
Operative time [min]	229	181	201	153.3
LOS [min]	99	142	240	2082
Ectopic pregnancy [%]	11	13	22	10
Complication rate [%]	3.8	14.6	5.5%	0%

Results are presented as mean, number [n] and percentages [%]. LOS: length of stay.

COMPLICATIONS OF ROBOTICS IN GYNECOLOGICAL ONCOLOGY

Robotic technology has revolutionized surgical treatment of gynecological cancers. Substantial magnification, dexterity, and flexibility offered by the robots simplify hysterectomy and pelvic lymphadenectomy. Boggess *et al* compared hysterectomy with staging for endometrial cancer using the robots, laparoscopy or laparotomy technique. They concluded that robotic assistance makes the lymphadenectomy and staging easier and comprehensive. They reported the overall complication rate of 6% for robots as compared to 11% for laparoscopy and 41% for laparotomy. The complications included bowel injury, port site hernia, lymphedema and vaginal leak [33].

Seamon *et al* in their experience with robotic hysterectomy and lymphadenectomy for endometrial cancers reported an overall complication rate of 13%. The complications included inferior vena cava injury, bowel injury, bowel obstruction, vaginal leak, pelvic abscess, and seroma in the midline port. They also reported fascial dehiscence after the extension of the midline port to remove a large uterus [34].

Magrina *et al* compared radical hysterectomy using robots, laparoscopy and laparotomy for cervical cancer. They reported the overall complication rate of 29% with robots, 22% with laparoscope and 31% with open technique. The robotic complications included bilateral pleural effusion, pneumothorax, urinary retention, urinary tract infection and lymphedema of lower extremity [35]. Boggess *et al* compared radical hysterectomy and lymph node dissection for cervical cancer with the robotic technique and the laparotomy. They found an overall complication rate of 7.8% in the robotic group and 16.3% in the laparotomy group. The robotic complication included cuff abscess, vaginal cuff dehiscence and lymph edema [36].

Nezhat also compared the robotic radical hysterectomy and lymphadenectomy to the conventional laparoscopic approach for treatment of early cervical cancer. They found the surgical outcomes of robotics similar to laparoscopy. They reported 4 complications in the robotic cases including ileus, urinary retention, vaginal lymph drainage and colitis [37].

COMPLICATIONS OF ROBOTICS IN SACROCOLPOPEXY

Abdominal sacrocolpopexy appears to be the most effective procedure for vaginal vault prolapse [38]. Technical difficulties and increased operative time with laparoscopic approach have limited its widespread use. The use of robot might overcome these difficulties. Elliott *et al* published their experience in robotically assisted laparoscopy for vaginal vault prolapse. They found similar durability of repair as with the open procedure but with minimum morbidity. Complications were limited to port site infections, recurrent rectocele and delayed erosion of the synthetic cuff into the vagina [39].

In another series, Daneshgari *et al* concluded that robotic abdominal sacrocolpopexy had favorable anatomic outcomes to the open and laparoscopic methods. They encountered one case of serosal bladder injury and another case of unresolved symptoms after the surgery [40]. The largest series is reported by Geller *et al* who compared the robotic sacrocolpopexy to the abdominal sacrocolpopexy. They reported similar short-term surgical outcomes with the robots with longer operative time. Complication rates were 19% in the robotic group and 15.2% in the abdominal group. The complications in the robotic group included pulmonary emboli, urinary tract injury, ileus, post operative fever and infections [41].

CONCLUSIONS

The use of surgical robot has given another venue to minimally invasive surgical options for women with gynecological disorders. To date, the literature consists of surgical techniques and short term clinical outcomes from investigators in their early learning experiences. Although improved perioperative outcomes appear to be associated with the robotic approach, randomized trials and well defined clinical studies with long term outcomes are needed to fully assess the value of this new technology.

REFERENCES

[1]   Chung SM, Jung YW, Lee SH, *et al.* Cost effective analysis of hysterectomy *via* laparotomy, laparoscopy and robotic assisted laparoscopy [Abstract] J Gynecol Oncol 2009; 20(Suppl 1): 150S.

[2]   Morgan JA, Thornton BA, Peacock JC, *et al.* Does robotic technology make minimal invasive cardiac surgery expensive? A hospital cost analysis of robotic and conventional techniques. J Card Surg 2005; 20: 246-251.

[3]   Lenihan JP, Kovanda C, Seshadri-Kreaden U. What is the learning curve for robotic assisted gynecologic surgery? J Minim Invasive Gynecol 2008; 15: 589-594.

[4]   Seamon LG, Fowler JM, Richardson DL, *et al.* A detailed analysis of the learning curve: robotic hysterectomy and pelvic-aortic lymphadenectomy for endometrial cancer. Gynecol Oncol 2009; 114: 162-167.

[5]   Altgassen C, Michels W, Schneider A. Learning laparoscopic-assisted hysterectomy. Obstet Gynecol 2004; 104: 308-313.

[6]   Kreiker GL, Bertoldi A, Larcher JS, *et al.* Prospective evaluation of the learning curve of laparoscopic-assisted vaginal hysterectomy in the university hospital. J Am Assoc Gynecol Laparosc 2004; 11: 229-235.

[7]   Tonouchi H, Ohmori Y, Kobayashi M. Trocar site hernia. Arch Surg 2004; 139: 1248-1256.

[8]   Seamon LG, Backers F, Resnick K, *et al.* Robotic trocar site small bowel evisceration after gynecological cancer surgery. Obstet Gynecol 2008; 112: 462-464.

[9]   Wu JM, Wechter ME, Geller EJ, *et al.* Hysterectomy rates in United States, 2003. Obstet Gynecol 2007; 110: 1091-5.

[10]   Johnson N, Barlow D, Lethaby A, *et al.* Methods of hysterectomy: Systemic review and meta-analysis of randomized controlled trials. BNJ 2005; 330: 1478.

[11]   Payne TN, Dauterive FR. A comparision of total laparoscopic hysterectomy to robotic assisted hysterectomy: Surgical outcomes in a community practice. J Minim Invasive Gynecol 2008; 15: 286-291.

[12]   Shashoua AR, Gill D, Locher SR. Robotica-assisted total laparoscopic hysterectomyversus conventional total laparoscopic hysterectomy. JSLS 2009; 13: 364-369.

[13]   Payne TN, Dauterive FR, Pitter MC, *et al.* Robotically assisted hysterectomy in patients with large uteri. Obstet Gynecol 2010; 115: 535-541.

[14]   Kho RM, Akl MN, Cornella JL *et al.* Incidence of characteristics of patients with vaginal cuff dehiscence after robotic procedures. Obstet Gynecol 2009; 114: 231-235.

[15]   Agdi M, Al-Ghafri W, Antolin R, Arrington J, O'Kelley K, Thomson AJM, O'Kelley K, Tulandi T. Vaginal vault dehiscence after hysterectomy. J Min Inv Gynecol 2009; 16: 313-7.

[16]   Holloway RW, Patel SD, Ahmad S. Robotic surgery in gynecology. Scand J Surg 2009; 98: 96-109.

[17]   Tomassetti C, Meuleman C, Vanacker B. Lower limb compartment syndrome as a complication of laparoscopic laser surgery for severe endometriosis. Fertil steril 2009; 92: 2038.e9-e12.

[18]   Beste TM, Nelson KH, Daucher JA. Total laparoscopic hysterectomy utilizing a robotic surgical system. JSLS 2005; 9: 13-15.

[19]   Fiorentino RP, Zepeda MA, Goldstien BH, *et al.* Pilot study assessing robotic laparoscopic hysterectomy and patient outcomes. J Minim Invasive Gynecol 2006; 13: 60-63.

[20]   Reynolds RK, Advincula AP. Robot-asiated laparoscopic hysterectomy: Technique and initial experience. Am J Surg 2006; 191: 555-560.

[21] Kho RM, Hilger WS, Hentz JG, *et al.* Robotic hysterectomy: Technique and initial outcomes. Am J Obstet Gynecol 2007; 197: 113.e1-e4.

[22] Lenihan JP Jr, Kovanda C, Seshardi-Kreaden U. What is the learning curve for robotic assisted surgery? J Minim Invasive Gynecol 2008; 15: 589-594.

[23] Boggess JF, Gehrig PA, Cantrell L, *et al.* Perioperative outcomes of robotically assisted hysterectomy for benign cases with complex pathology. Obstet Gynecol 2009; 114: 585-593.

[24] Nezhat C, Lavie O, Lemyre M, *et al.* Laparoscopic hysterectomy with and without a robot: Stanford experience. JSLS 2009; 13: 125-128.

[25] Falcone T, Bedaiwy MA. Minimally invasive management of uterine fibroids. Cur Opin Obstet Gynecol 2002; 14: 401-407.

[26] Advincula AP, Xu X, Goudeau S, *et al.* Robotic assisted laparoscopic myomectomy versus abdominal myomectomy: A comparison of short-term surgical outcomes and immediate costs. J Minim Invasive Gynecol 2007; 14: 698-705.

[27] Nezhat C, Lavie O, Hsu S, *et al.* Robotic-assisted laparoscopic myoomectomy compared with standard laparoscopic myomectomy- a retrospective matched control study. Fertil Steril 2009; 91: 556-559.

[28] Bedient CE, Magrina JF, Noble BN, *et al.* Comparison of robotic and laparoscopic myomectomy. A J Obstet Gynecol 2009; 201: 566.e1-5.

[29] George A, Eisenstein D, Wegienka G. Analysis of the impact of body mass index on the surgical outcomes after robot-asisted laparoscopic myomectomy. J Minim Invasive Gynecol 2009; 16: 730-733.

[30] Degueldre M, Vandromme J, Huong PT, *et al.* Robotic assisted laparoscopic microsurgical tubal reanastomosis: a feasibility study. Fertil Steril 2000; 74: 1020-1023.

[31] Rodgers AK, Goldberg JM, Hammel JP, *et al.* Tubal anastomosis by robotic compared with outpatient minilaparotomy. Obstet Gynecol 2007; 109: 1375-1380.

[32] Dharia Patel SP, Steinkampf MP, Whitten SJ, *et al.* Robotic tubal anastomosis: surgical technique and cost effectiveness. Fertil steril 2008; 90: 1175-1179.

[33] Boggess JF, Gehrig PA, Cantrell L, *et al.* A comparative study of 3 surgical methods for hysterectomy with staging for endometrial cancer: robotic assistance, laparoscopy, laparotomy. Am J Obstet Gynecol 2008; 199: 360 e1-360e9.

[34] Seamon LG, Cohn DE, Richardson DL, *et al.* Robotic hysterectomy and pelvic-aortic lymphadenectomy for endometrial cancer. Obstet Gynecol 2008; 112: 1207-1213.

[35] Magrina JF, Kho RM, Weaver AL, *et al.* Robotic radical hysterectomy: Comparison with laparoscopy and laparotomy. Gynecol Oncol 2008; 109: 86-91.

[36] Boggess JF, Gehrig PA, Cantrell L, *et al.* A case-control study of robot-assisted type III radical hysterectomy with pelvic lymph node dissection compared with open radical hysterectomy. Am J Obstet Gynecol 2008; 199: 357e1-357e7.

[37] Nezhat FR, Datta MS, Liu C, *et al.* Robotic radical hysterectomy versus total laparoscopic radical hysterectomy with pelvic lymphadenectomy for treatment of early cervical cancer. JSLS 2008; 12: 227-237.

[38] Timmons MC, Addison WA, Addison SB, *et al.* Abdominal sacralcolpopexy in 163 women with posthyaterectomy vaginal vault prolapse and enterocele. J Reprod Med 1992 1992; 37: 323-327.

[39] Elliott DS, Frank I, DiMarco DS, *et al.* Gynecological use of robotically assisted laparoscopy: sacrocolpopexy for the treatment of high grade vaginal vault prolapse. Am J Surg 2004; 188: 52S-56S.

[40] Daneshgari F, Kefer JC, Moore C, *et al.* Robotic abdominal sacrocolpopexy/sacrouteropexy repair of advanced female pelvic organ prolapse [POP]: utilizing POP-quantification-based staging and outcomes. BJU Int 2007; 100: 875-879.

[41] Geller EJ, Siddiqui NY, Wu JM, *et al.* Short-term outcomes of robotic sacrocolpopexy compared with abdominal sacrocolpopexy. Obstet Gynecol 2008; 112: 1201-1206.

CHAPTER 8

Avoiding Complications in Robotic Surgery in Gynecology

Rosanne M. Kho*

Division of Urogynecology and Pelvic Reconstructive Surgery, Department of Gynecologic Surgery, Mayo Clinic AZ, 5777 E Mayo Blvd, Phoenix, AZ 85057, USA

Abstract: Robotics surgery differs from conventional laparoscopy in the absence of tactile feedback, need to perform procedure remotely and presence of fixed and rigid robotic arms. These factors bring a unique set of considerations that need to be recognized in order to avoid complications.

INTRODUCTION

The robotic surgical system is increasingly applied to all aspects of gynecologic surgery including general gynecology, reproductive, urogynecology and gynecologic oncology [1]. With widespread use, complications unique to the robotic approach are identified [2]. The following chapter reviews factors that contribute to complications in robotics in gynecologic procedures and discusses recommendations on how complications can be avoided.

FACTORS THAT CONTRIBUTE TO COMPLICATIONS IN ROBOTICS

All complications associated with conventional laparoscopic surgery could be encountered with robotics surgery. Though the robotic surgical system provides multiple advantages over conventional laparoscopy such as 3D-imaging, instrument articulation and down-scaling of movements, other factors such as lack of tactile feedback, need to perform procedure remotely [*i.e.*, not at the patient's bedside], and the fixed and rigid positions of the robotic arms can bring upon a set of complications that are unique to robotics.

A. Lack of Tactile Feedback

The current robotic surgical system does not provide haptics. Reliance on visual cues is paramount when there is absence of immediate and direct tactile feedback. Visual cues such as blanching of the tissue when traction is applied or 'give' of the tissue when pressure is applied are valuable signs for the robotic surgeon. The surgeon should give attention to the amount of traction provided by the grasping instrument [on the non-dominant hand] to avoid unnecessary bleeding and oozing. It is our experience that bleeding more often occurs from excessive traction provided by the grasping rather than the dissecting instrument.

Lack of haptics necessitate that robotic instruments are moved only under direct visualization to avoid inadvertent injury to important intra-abdominal structures. In the event that the surgeon is unable to locate a robotic instrument, the bedside assistant can bring this back into view by un-clutching the robotic arm and bringing the instrument back to the surgeon's visual field.

The use of a '4th' arm is also unique to the robotics approach. This arm remains fixed in its position until activated at the console by the robotic surgeon. A grasping instrument to retract tissues is the favored instrument for the 4th arm. Though use of the 4th arm can greatly facilitate the procedure, there is a learning curve involved in its use. Placement of the 4th arm trocar on the abdominal wall should be carefully planned to avoid arm collisions with the ipsilateral robotic arm. The 4th arm trocar should be positioned 10cm lateral and inferior to the right or left robotic trocar [depending on the planned procedure] to avoid arm collision Fig. **1**. In the majority of our gynecologic procedures, the bedside assistant is seated at the patient's left side with the accessory trocar positioned on the patient's left upper

*Address correspondence to Dr. Rosanne Kho: Department of Gynecologic Surgery, Mayo Clinic AZ, 5777 E Mayo Blvd, Phoenix AZ 85057, USA. Email: kho.rosanne@mayo.edu

quadrant. The 4th arm in these cases is therefore positioned on the patient's right. Occasionally, such as in a sacrocolpopexy, the 4th arm is positioned on the patient's left side in order to retract the sigmoid colon laterally. In this situation, the accessory trocar is positioned on the patient's right. Arm collisions between the ipsilateral and 4th arms can inadvertently cause injury to important intra-abdominal structures such as large vessels and bowel. Because the 4th arm is often used for retraction and is out of the surgeon's view, the instrument on the 4th arm should therefore never be used to directly retract vessels such as the external or internal iliac vessels. Instead, retraction can be accomplished by grasping the peritoneum overlying important structures, or indirectly by *tucking the structure behind opened jaws* Box **1**.

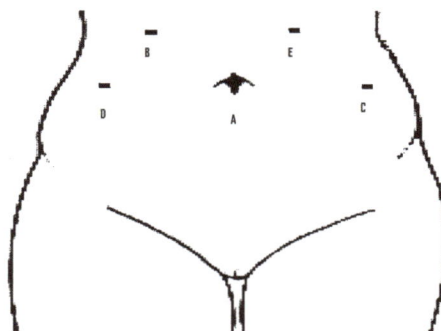

Figure 1: Trocar placement showing "M" configuration. [A- umbilical port for robotic scope; In majority of cases, B and C- lateral 8 mm robotic trocars; D - 4th arm, E - 10 mm accessory port. In sacrocolpopexy, E and D – lateral 8 mm ports, C – 4th arm, B – accessory port.]

Summary Box 1:

> a.   *Possible complications due to lack of tactile feedback:*
>   i.   *Bleeding from undue traction and pressure*
>   ii. *Movement of instruments outside of the surgeon's visual field [such as the 4th arm instrument] can injure intra-abdominal structures.*
> b.   *To avoid the above complications:*
>   i.   *Attention to visual cues*
>   ii. *Do not move robotic instruments that are outside of the surgeon's visual field.*

B. Remote Performance of Procedure

Performance of the procedure while seated remotely at the robotic console is a unique feature to the robotic surgical approach. A dedicated robotic bedside team is critical in facilitating safe and efficient surgery. Effective and continual communication between the surgeon at the console and the bedside team is necessary to avoid complications. In our practice, the bedside team includes the surgical assistant [seated at the patient's left] and scrub nurse [seated at the patient's right]. Important roles of the robotic bedside team include:

a.   Maintenance of sterility at the patient's bedside to minimize risks for infection and pelvic abscess. Organizing cords and tubings with blue towels and clips can be helpful to avoid contamination. It is important that the drapes on the robotic arms do not brush against non-sterile surfaces [such as the intravenous pole or the assistant's mask]. When this occurs, a large sterile tape [such as Tagaderm, 3M] can be placed over the contaminated area to avoid re-draping.

Tracking of suture needles. An accessory port [10-12 mm trocar] is placed so that the assistant can insert and retrieve sutures [with CT-1 or CT-2 needles] easily through this port. In case of a needle lost within the abdomen during needle retrieval, the needle is often found directly below the trocar or overlying the omentum or loops of bowel. It is important not to take the patient out of Trendelenberg or move the loops of bowel to search for the lost needle.

b.   Ensuring robotic arm mobility. Arm movements can be limited by arm collision and also by the plastic drapes that stick to the distal portion of the robotic arm. Confirming that the elbows of the robotic arms are at least a fist-size apart from each other at the beginning of the case and that the sterile drapes overlying each arm remain loose at all times can facilitate safety.

c.   Making sure that the robotic arms, particularly the most lateral or caudal arms do not impinge upon patient's extremities [arms/hands, thighs/feet] at any point during surgery.

Summary Box 2:

> *Possible complications due to performance of procedure remotely necessitate reliance on the bedside team:*
> *a.   Loss of sterility that can lead to infection*
> *b.   Lost needles that can be difficult to find*
> *c.   Limited mobility of robotic arms*
> *d.   Injury to patient's extremities*

C. Fixed and Rigid Robotic Arms

In contrast to conventional laparoscopy, robotic trocars are held in a fixed and rigid position by the robotic arms. In pelvic surgery where steep [30°] Trendelenberg is necessary, it is important that the patient is safely positioned without risk of sudden shifting or sliding during the surgery. We recommend the use of an anti-skid material [such as the eggcrate foam] taped securely to the table Fig. **2**. The patient lays on her bare back directly on the foam material while the arms are tucked to the side and legs positioned in the modified dorsal lithotomy position using the Yellofin stirrups [Allen Medical, MA]. Ensuring a large surface area of the patient's back against the anti-skid material ensures ample friction and prevents sliding. We do not recommend the use of straps, braces or shoulder blocks to avoid a neuropathy. Our study has shown that this technique is safe and effectively minimizes sliding during Trendelenberg [3].

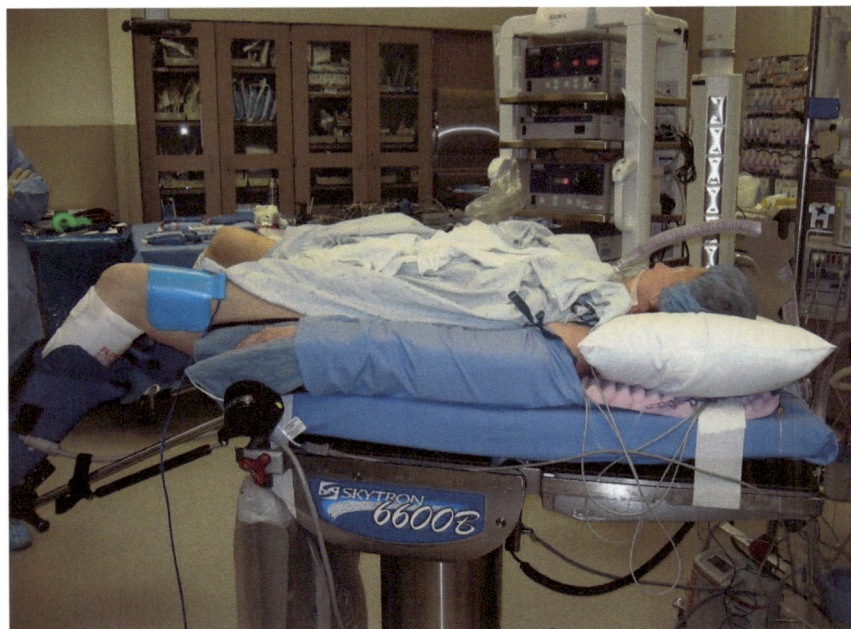

Figure 2: Anti-skid material is used with proper patient positioning to prevent patient shifting during steep Trendelenberg.

Because robotic trocars are held in a rigid fixed position, loss of pneumoperitoneum could result in not only loss of visualization but also collapse of the abdominal wall and subsequent dislodgement of the robotic trocars. It is important therefore to maintain constant pneumoperitoneum during robotic surgery. This can be achieved by gently squeezing the labia during colpotomy and insertion of a balloon vaginal occluder [Colpo-pneumo occluder, Cooper Surgical, CT] during vaginal cuff closure.

D. 8 mm Port Site Hernia

Port site hernia from the 8 mm trocars happens infrequently and can be minimized with the use of the blunt or bladeless obturators available Fig. **3**. We do not recommend routine fascial closure of the 8 mm port but consider it when significant manipulation is applied through this site resulting in fascial stretching.

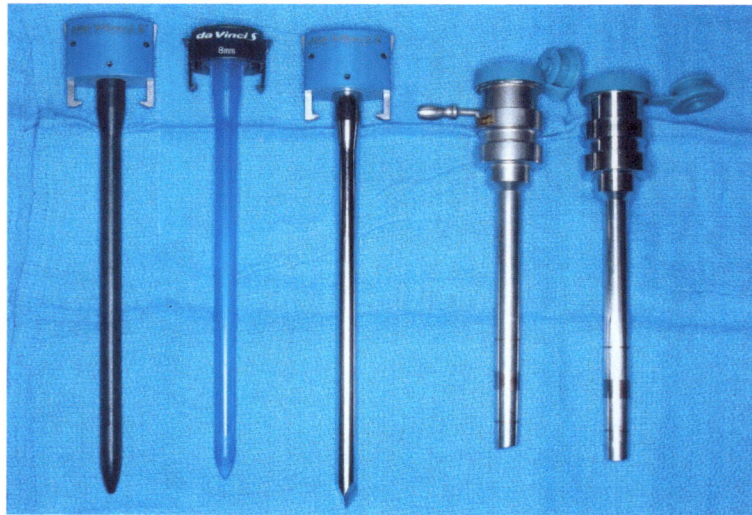

Figure 3: Blunt or bladeless trocars [first and second from the right] are preferred to minimize fascial defects.

E. Electrocoagulation and Vaginal Cuff Dehiscence

Vaginal cuff dehiscence is rare but can occur after robotic procedures [4]. The reported incidence of 4.1% is similar to the laparoscopic approach at 4.9% [5]. In our experience, patients with vaginal cuff dehiscence after a robotic procedure presented at a mean time of 7 weeks after the procedure. This event occurred spontaneously or was triggered by coitus. It is important that patients who present with sudden onset of vaginal bleeding or gush of watery discharge even beyond the 6-week post-operative period are brought in immediately for an examination.

Electrocoagulation use during colpotomy, which is unique to the laparoscopic and robotic approaches, more than likely contributes a significant factor in the delay of tissue healing. It should be noted that because recurrence of dehiscence can occur unless vaginal edges are trimmed with cold knife further suggests that the electrocoagulation can have long lasting effects on tissue healing.

Prevention of vaginal cuff dehiscence in robotics can be achieved by minimizing use of extensive electrocoagulation during colpotomy. Colpotomy can be primarily accomplished using cut-mode set at 35 watts. Limited spot coagulation using coagulation-mode can be performed to achieve hemostasis. The vaginal cuff is closed with full-thickness purchase of the cuff tissue incorporating both the anterior and posterior fascia that is at least 5 mm beyond the coagulated edge. Additional preventive measures include a 2-layer closure of the cuff, either with additional figure-of-eight stitches or with a running suture, and with the use of a delayed-absorbable suture such as polydiaxanone [PDS, Ethicon].

In the event of bowel evisceration with the dehiscence, a large sterile wet lapatotomy sponge is used to wrap and protect the loops of bowel while mobilizing the operating room team. Intravenous antibiotics for gram-positive coverage is initiated. Under anesthesia and with the patient in dorsal lithotomy position, the loops of bowel are copiously irrigated before reducing back into the abdominal cavity. This is achieved vaginally with the surgeon's fingers instead of traumatic instruments. Once reduced, the bladder is mobilized from the anterior vaginal cuff edge and the rectum from the posterior. At least 1 cm of the vaginal cuff edge is trimmed with a scalpel or with cold scissors to 'freshen' the edges and minimize the risk of a recurrent dehiscence. The vaginal cuff is reapproximated using interrupted sutures. Prior to closure of the vaginal cuff, we recommend running the bowel proximally and distally to ensure viability. None of the patients in our series with bowel evisceration required bowel resection Box **3**.

Summary Box 3:

Measures to prevent vaginal cuff dehiscence:
  a. *full-thickness purchase of anterior and posterior vaginal cuff that is at least 5 mm beyond the coagulated edge*
  b. *avoid extensive electrocoagulation during colpotomy*
  c. *perform a second layer closure with additional figure-of-eight or running suture*

REFERENCES

[1]   Visco AG, Advincula AP. Robotic gynecologic surgery. Obstet Gynecol 2008; 112: 1369.

[2]   Giles DL, Long JB, Akl MN, *et al.* 500 robotic surgical cases for benign and oncologic conditions in gynecology. Poster. Society of Gynecologic Surgery Annual Scientific Meeting. April 14-16, 2008. Savannah, GA.

[3]   Klauschie J, Wechter ME, Jacob K, *et al.* Use of Anti-skid material and patient-positioning to prevent patient shifting during robotic-assisted gynecologic procedures. J Minim Invasive Gynecol 2010; 17(4): 504-7.

[4]   Kho RM, Akl MN, Cornella JL, Magtibay PM, Wechter ME, Magrina JF. Incidence and characteristics of patients with vaginal cuff dehiscence after robotic procedures. Obstet Gynecol 2009; 114: 231.

[5]   Hur HC, Guido RS, Mansuria SM, *et al.* Incidence and patient characteristics of vaginal cuff dehiscence after different modes of hysterectomies. J Minim Invasive Gynecol 2007; 14: 311.

Index

A

Aesop, 4

B

Cervical cancer, 54
Cervicosacropexy, 10, 16
Classification of hysterectomy, 30
Colposacropexy, 10, 12
Colpotomy, 37
Complication, 62, 69

D

DaVinci, 5
Dehiscence, 72, 73
Dual surgeon console, 5

E

Endometrial cancer results, 51-53
Endometrial cancer, 50
Endowrist, 8, 23

G

Gynecologic oncology complication, 66

H

Hermes, 4
Hernia, 72
History, 3, 28, 41
Hysterectomy complication, 64
Hysterectomy results, 39
Hysterectomy, 27, 63

L

Limitation, 22, 62

M

Myomectomy complication, 64-65
Myomectomy results, 21
Myomectomy results, 65
Myomectomy, 17

N

Nodal dissection, 55-56

O

Ovarian cancer, 57

P

Pelvic exenteration, 56
Port placement , 11, 23, 31-33, 44
Positioning, 23, 31, 43, 71

R

Radical hysterectomy, 54
Radical trachelectomy, 55
Robotic vs. conventional laparoscopic myomectomy, 21

S

Sacrocolpopexy complications, 66
Sacrocolpopexy, 10-12
Set-up, 23, 30
Socrates, 5

T

Technique of hysterectomy, 29
Trocar placement , 11, 23, 31-33, 44, 70
Trocars, 72
Tubal anastomosis results, 43
Tubal anastomosis technique, 44
Tubal anastomosis, 41
Tubal anastomosis, 65-66

Z

Zeus, 4